The Cancer Companion

A guide to getting your head and heart around your diagnosis and treatment

BY SARAH E. MCDONALD

The Cancer Companion

Published by:

Sarah McDonald Press
sarahemcdonald.com

Second Edition

Printed in the United States of America
ISBN: 978-1-958777-06-0 (paperback)
ISBN: 978-1-958777-07-7 (eBook)

Neither the publisher nor the author is engaged in rendering professional advice or services to the individual reader. This book is not intended for use as a source of health, medical, legal, or financial advice. All readers are advised to seek the services of competent professionals in the health, medical, legal, and financial fields. Neither the author nor the publisher shall be liable or responsible for any loss or damage allegedly arising from any information or suggestions in this book.

While the author has made every effort to provide accurate internet addresses at the time of publication, neither the publisher nor the author assumes any responsibility for errors or for changes that occur after publication. Further, the publisher does not have any control over and does not assume any responsibility for third-party websites or their content.

To Tripti for being in charge of Team Two and for teaching me to breathe through this

---

To Geoff and Rory for always being on my team. I choose you.

"I know God will not give me anything I can't handle. I just wish He didn't trust me so much."

_____

-- MOTHER TERESA

Table of Contents

Introduction

I know it might feel this way right now, but you're not alone.

I was forty-four when I was diagnosed with a rare, incurable cancer called adenoid cystic carcinoma (salivary gland cancer). The diagnosing doctor read the survival statistics to me from a website. "After five years, 80% of people are still alive. After ten years, it drops to 30%."

Those statistics literally took my breath away. I was stunned. I was terrified. I didn't know – really – what I should do. And I felt completely alone.

Who could I turn to? Who was going to help me? No one I knew, who was my age at least, had cancer. I didn't know where I should be getting my information (the doctor was reading from a website on the internet?!?).

The medical professionals I was trying to see had long waiting lists, with some backed up for three months or more. It seemed surreal to be told I had cancer, but then be expected to wait in terror for my turn to be told how it might be treated (or not). I was reeling and felt like I had no one to help me navigate this life-altering news.

And then I got a second, totally unrelated cancer diagnosis. This one was called invasive ductal carcinoma or, as I would come to know it, breast cancer. Stage 3.

I was completely at a loss. The fear I felt was beyond anything I had ever experienced before. I tried to get my head around my diagnoses. And I was desperate to learn about my prognosis. I worried about the future, and perhaps more to the point, if I would have a future.

So, I turned to the library. I read every book I could find on why cancer happens, what treatments were available for my cancers, and what I might expect (side effects) from my cancer treatment plans. These books were written by doctors. I learned a lot about the science and physicality of cancer; what was happening to my body and why.

And while I appreciated what I learned from the doctors who wrote those books, I needed information that went beyond the physical. I needed someone who could talk with me about the emotional aspects of my cancer diagnosis. I needed someone to tell me it was okay that I was freaking out – or to tell me how to stop freaking out. I needed someone who knew the hacks for the side effects I might experience. What I needed was a guide. Or better yet, a guidebook...a "how-to" manual for cancer.

But I didn't find one. So, I wrote one based upon what I learned. I tried to speak to the questions I had during my first days/weeks/months of understanding what it meant to be living with cancer.

I'd love to tell you that this book answers ALL of your potential questions about your cancer, but it won't. I've had two cancers so I'm not a total novice, but the reality is that every cancer type is different (there are over 200 cancers out there!). And every person's journey is unique. I'm not going to be able address every nuance of every cancer, or your particular circumstances. I'm just not. And I am truly sorry for that.

My goal with this book is to help you start to get your head around your diagnosis and provide you some guidance on your journey. It's the stuff I would speak with you about if we met and had coffee (or, probably more appropriately, a cocktail or a whole bottle of wine) together. It is a high-level overview of cancer – a starting point on your journey.

I am so very sorry you are going through this. I know it must be hard. These pages are designed to help you better understand the issues and possible scenarios you will encounter as you begin mapping out plans to overcome this disease. I am not here to tell you how to "do" cancer, I am simply hopeful that this book makes your journey a little easier...

May you be happy

May you be healthy

May you be at peace

Sarah

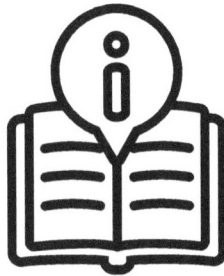

Chapter 01

How are You Doing?
No, Really.

Even if you suspected something was wrong in your body, even if you were the one who found your cancer, I'm not sure anyone is prepared to hear the words "You have cancer." It is unmooring. And really, if we're being honest about it, unbelievable. You've always been pretty healthy, right?

And now...*this*.

And it is scary.

And it can be lonely.

And it requires things of you that you never imagined before.

Cancer requires a fluency in a totally new (medical) language that includes words like "prognosis" and "perineural invasion." It requires knowledge of treatment options, side effects, and clinical trials. It can often require a ninja-level ability to manage tests, scans, appointments, and medications. And that's just on the medical front.

Newly-diagnosed cancer patients also have to figure out how to communicate this scary health news with family and friends, not to mention their employer and work teammates. And it would be one thing if cancer was a comfortable topic for (most) people to discuss, but it is not. People whisper about cancer, afraid perhaps that if they speak in a natural voice cancer will come after them? (This is when I try to remind people that cancer is not contagious.)

AND wouldn't it be great if the treatment of (and survival from) cancer followed a predictable path that everyone was familiar with? But it does not. It turns out that every *body* is different, and so, different bodies respond differently to cancer AND, perhaps not surprising, every *body* responds differently to cancer treatments. Some work. Some do not. Treatment plans (and our body's reaction to them) vary greatly.

So how do you communicate to people when it is a topic they're afraid to speak of AND when the outcome is unpredictable? And when you don't have all the answers and are freaking out?

It is simply a lot. A cancer diagnosis is A LOT.

I call out all of these things not to add to your overwhelm, but rather to justify (for you, for others) the overwhelm you might be feeling. It is totally normal to feel fear, anxiety, panic, anger, denial, sadness, and bewilderment. These are all typical (and acceptable!) feelings associated with receiving shocking (and perhaps devastating) health news.

The Cancer Companion

Please note that if you read the above list of challenges and you aren't freaking out – well, then either you have an amazing meditation practice or you are (or may be) in denial. Either way, I am glad you're not freaking out. The rest of us are.

I want to start this simple guidebook with an acknowledgement of the four-alarm panic you might be feeling right now. I want to assure you that you are normal for feeling like you're losing your mind. It is okay to feel all of these feelings, deeply. No matter what kind of cancer you have, you are justified in feeling anxiety, grief, and overwhelm. They said the word "CANCER" to you, right?

You have cancer. It is now a part of your life story. Hopefully a small part, but a part. You don't know (and can't control) how that story will play out. In fact, you won't be able to control a lot of what happens next. But I'm going to share with you what I learned, often the hard way, on practical ways to manage those parts of your cancer diagnosis, treatment, and story you can control.

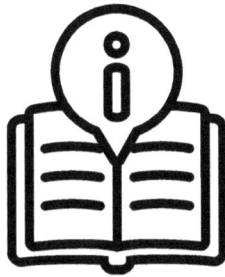

Chapter 02

Ideas for How Not to Lose Your Mind

The Cancer Companion

Yes, cancer is a physical disease and the treatment for cancer can be physically challenging. But it can also be a mental and emotional struggle. For many of us, it is the first time we are coming face-to-face with the reality of our own mortality. And that can be life-altering. Mind-bending. Terror-inducing.

For me, the mental and emotional toll was harder than any of the more tangible physical side effects that plagued my body. That is telling, since I lost thirty-five pounds because I couldn't eat for three weeks. This was due to concurrent radiation and chemotherapy treatments that resulted in seventeen cold sores erupting in what felt like a sunburned mouth. Yep, I counted them. It gave me something better to focus on than the pain for a few moments. Seriously.

Physically, I was a wreck. Mentally and emotionally, I was worse.

It was rough, but I made it through my cancer treatments physically, mentally, and emotionally by focusing on calming my anxiety. I would suggest you try anything and everything you can, but here are some (gentle) starting suggestions:

Create Space in Your Calendar (if you can)

Allow yourself some space to process this big news – at least in the initial days and weeks. Yes, you are in the midst of a health crisis, but you likely aren't going to die tomorrow. At least not from the cancer. Create time and space on your calendar for processing this important health news. I know this makes me sound like I'm from Northern California (I am) but honestly, your cancer diagnosis is a big deal. At the very least, you're going to have to find time over the next couple of weeks or months for doctor appointments, possible surgery, and potential other treatments. This is a time to get comfortable with prioritizing your physical and mental health above all other commitments.

It's Okay to Freak Out, but Don't Make Major Life Decisions Right Now

It is okay to cry and/or scream and/or beat your pillow. If you need permission to do any of those things, you have it. But given that your life has been turned upside down (and you may not even recognize it or, frankly, yourself right now), this is not the time to make major life decisions. A cancer diagnosis changes your life in ways big and small that you don't even know yet.

I have one friend who (in a fit of freakout) quit his job the day after his cancer diagnosis. This decision certainly gave him more time to process his diagnosis and go to appointments, but it also left him without health insurance. This added a self-induced (and very stressful) financial component to his cancer treatment! Ugh.

You don't know what your cancer journey will look like. No one does. So please don't make major decisions about your life based upon information you don't have. It is an uncomfortable place to be, this place of "not knowing," but perhaps it is better to sit with "not knowing" than it is to dive headfirst into damage control for the rash decision(s) you made when you were out of your head with cancer-diagnosis-panic.

It Is Okay (and Normal) to Mourn

While it is difficult to say out loud, the future you expected for yourself was never guaranteed. It has been altered and perhaps even lost. That is a lot to process. The processing of this major change can feel a whole lot like grief...because it is grief. It is loss of your imagined future.

My first cancer diagnosis came sixteen months after my wedding to my husband Geoff, four months after I had received a major promotion at work, and *one week* before I was scheduled for invitro-fertilization (IVF) with plans to start a family. I had big dreams for what my life was going to become. Suddenly I felt it all being ripped away from me with the words, "You have cancer." Instead of dreams, I was now living in a nightmare.

Grief is non-linear. It has no timeline. And it has no rules. AND it is different for each person. It can soften and lessen with time as you become used to the word cancer being associated with you, but I suspect it will stay with you, as it does for most people I've met.

A friend of mine, who is a clinical psychologist, tells me that one of the most unhelpful things people can do to themselves when they are in grief is to impose a timeline on their grief or tell themselves *how* they should grieve. Grief is going to take the time it is going to take. You are going to feel what you are going to feel. Give yourself some (maybe a lot of) grace and let yourself feel all of the feels right now.

Breathe into and Accept (as best you can) the Not-knowing

Dr. Seuss wrote a terrific, much-celebrated book called "Oh, the places you'll go!" His message focuses on the journey of life and how it will be filled with wonderful adventures *and* difficulties. His encouragement to try new things and be resilient are inspirational, making this book one that is regularly gifted at graduations as young people embark on adulting. *And* he shares with the reader the challenges of places they'll encounter on their life journey that will be really hard such as the "waiting place" where everyone is standing around waiting for the next thing.

Unfortunately, a cancer diagnosis lands you firmly in that awful waiting place. You will find yourself waiting for appointments and waiting for scan and test results and waiting to hear of your treatment plan and waiting to hear what your prognosis is. It is a lot of waiting. And it is a lot of stuff that is out of your control. And it is a lot of not knowing.

It is enough to drive you crazy. This is the mental part of the diagnosis I mentioned before. And I found it to be the hardest part. It drove me to a level of panic and anxiety I had never experienced before. I call it out here so that you know you are not alone in feeling this way.

Here are some more ideas that might help soften your cancer-diagnosis-panic and anxiety:

Try Guided Imagery (and other Eastern practices)

When I was first diagnosed with cancer, one of my doctors recommended I check out something called **Guided Imagery.** I was not someone who did yoga or meditation so was a little skeptical of what I imagined to be a "woo woo" practice. But I agreed to check it out.

A quick Google search on guided imagery reveals it is "a form of focused relaxation that helps create harmony between the mind and body. It is a way of focusing your imagination to create calm, peaceful images in your mind, thereby providing a 'mental escape.'"

For the first two to three months of my cancer treatments, I listened to a guided imagery CD *at least* once day. I would sit on the floor of my bedroom, close my eyes, and hit the play button. A calm voice came on that encouraged me to walk in my mind's eye to a place I loved and to look around, see the grass or the water or the trees, feel the breeze. I settled on a walk through a small forest between Bay Beach and Slim Point at Silver Bay, New York; a place from my childhood.

I walked from the grassy patches of Bay Beach down to the rutted walkway that leads into the white birch woodland. There, among the imagined trees, I started crying. This was not the kind of crying where gentle, sweet tears run down your face. This was the wracking, snot-releasing sob of crying where animal sounds escape from your throat. I could not remain seated against the bed. I had to get up on my knees and then lean over to allow the sobs to work their way through me.

I have no idea why or how this guided-imagery worked, but wow, was it the catharsis I needed. I cried each time I listened to it. Alone. On my knees. Doubled over. Until one day...the stress released. I didn't wake up with my body tensed and my brain racing to figure out how to escape. Some kind of mind-body magic happened and I just relaxed. Now I constantly recommend Guided Imagery to others.

Get out and MOVE (if you can)

Exercise boosts your immune system, lifts your mood (endorphins!), strengthens your body, helps you sleep, and probably about seventeen other "good for you" things, including distracting you from thinking about cancer. This is a great time (Yes! Right now, when you've been diagnosed with cancer!) to start a regular exercise habit if you can.

This *does not* mean you need to start a running habit that would resemble training for a marathon. It means simply getting out and moving your body. That can certainly mean running, but it could also be walking or dancing. It can mean yoga, or Pilates, or just plain old stretching. You will be amazed how much your body will appreciate you taking the time to stretch it. I have found that stretching puts me in better tune with my body, more aware of which parts have pain (or not). This is especially true when I am wholly focused on my body for a timebound ten to fifteen minutes.

I believe that this practice of checking in with my body when it was undergoing cancer treatments was super helpful in building my confidence in my body. By running or doing yoga, I felt myself growing stronger. This was encouraging when I feared chemotherapy would weaken me. Walking on the cool sands of a beach allowed me to relax. The ocean air (and ginger throat lozenges) helped to keep my nausea in check. By stretching, I felt my body become more limber and I thanked it for all of the work it was doing to get rid of the cancer.

Breathe

Preferably in nature. But really anywhere that allows you to focus on breathing deeply and relaxing as best you can. Taking long breaths in and out actually calms the amygdala of your brain, which is the part of the brain that triggers the fight/flight/freeze reaction. Regardless of which of those reactions you're currently having (I'm a "flight" girl myself; my brain screams "RUN AWAY!"), the more you can breathe and calm your amygdala, the better both your mind and body will feel. Ideally, your cancer-diagnosis-panic will quiet down to a dull roar and you will begin to be able to think more clearly again. As your anxiety quiets, you will be better able to learn about, and plan for, your cancer treatment with your doctors.

A plan is a very good thing to have. It helps you see the path you and your medical team will take to try to rid your body of this horrible disease. A plan will help you feel like you are *doing something* about your cancer.

My hope is that it will help you breathe easier through all of this.

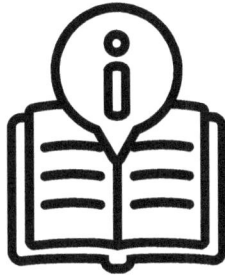

Chapter 03

You Have Cancer.
Now What?

The Cancer Companion

The American Cancer Society tells us that one in three women will be diagnosed with cancer during her lifetime. For men, it is one in two.

This is an alarming statistic. Especially now that it directly impacts YOU.

Ugh. So where should you start? Below are some gentle suggestions.

Learn Everything You Can About Your Cancer

Unless you have had a family member or close friend diagnosed with cancer, most people know very little about cancer until they receive a diagnosis themselves. My father was diagnosed with (prostate) cancer a decade before I received my cancer news, but I didn't *really dig in* until the "You have cancer" words were directed at me. What I discovered quickly is learning as much as I could about my cancer made me the best, most informed patient possible for my doctors. In practice, your doctors may actually ask for your input on treatment decisions so it is a good idea to have some idea of what the options are. In turn, being a well-informed patient who can effectively communicate issues, symptoms, and preferences gives doctors the opportunity to be the best, most informed doctors possible for you.

Here is a list of some of the basic questions you might ask your doctors about your cancer:

- ⋛ What kind of cancer is it?
    - ▶ Note: There are even subtypes within types of cancer.
- ⋛ What stage are you in?
    - ▶ Translated: How advanced is the cancer?
    - ▶ Is the cancer localized (just in one place) or has it moved into other organs (metastasized)?
- ⋛ How aggressive is this cancer?
    - ▶ Translated: How quickly are your cancer cells replicating and spreading?
    - ▶ Note: This will impact which treatment plan (think timeline and intensity) your doctors choose to recommend/pursue.
- ⋛ What treatments are available to you?
    - ▶ Depending on the type of cancer you have, there might be different cancer treatment plans ("protocols") that are recommended.
    - ▶ Note: Different cancers respond to different treatments.

For example, the chemotherapy given for breast cancer is different from chemotherapy given for prostate cancer. Still other cancers don't yet have a chemotherapy that works on them.

≳ What is your prognosis?

▶ Translated: What is your doctor's best guess as to what your health outcome will be?

▶ Note: This might also change over time if your body responds well (or doesn't) to the treatment plan.

Start Keeping a Log of Your Doctor Appointments/Scans/Tests

It is never too early to start taking notes. Take notes on what your doctors are telling you so that you can keep on top of the information (and understand it more fully). Document when you have a scan or a test and what the outcome is. Believe it or not, as you progress with treatments, appointments/scans/tests will all begin to blur together.

Yes, your medical center will have records of when a test or a scan was given, and you can cross-reference the radiologist's analysis of the test. But if you keep an ongoing log of your appointments and what was discussed, you'll have an easier time remembering, for example, why the doctor thought it was a good idea to do a follow up CT scan. It will help you have information at your fingertips concerning the last time you had an MRI. It will also allow you to keep track of which doctor said what. This can be helpful to your doctors. It will help inform your treatment decisions. I am a big fan of Excel spreadsheets, but a Word document or an old-fashioned written journal can work too. You should feel free to use whatever medium is most convenient, clear, and comforting to you.

Get a Second Opinion, Maybe a Third

This is a hard concept to consider when all you want to do is get the damned cancer out of you. A cancer diagnosis can drive a tremendous sense of urgency. This makes it hard to resist simply following whatever the first doctor tells you to do. But doctors sometimes differ in their opinions and treatment advice. It often makes sense to bring your scans and tests (and notes!) to another doctor to ask his/her opinion. Getting a second or even a third opinion is pretty standard practice. It will allow you to compare treatment options and determine what will work best for you as you continue to live your life. Yes, your quality of life as you go through cancer treatment is one of the things you and your doctors should consider.

Delaying your cancer treatment a week or two while you talk with other providers is usually okay (again, you are not dying tomorrow). If it means you find the right providers and right treatment for you, then it is worth it. Which brings us to the next topic...

Be Sure You Like and Trust Your Doctors

You are going to spend a lot of time with your doctors over the course of your treatments. You will want to be confident your doctors are committed to fighting on your behalf and will listen to you. Getting that second (or third) opinion provides you the opportunity to compare doctors (their assessment of your case, their suggested treatments, and perhaps most importantly, *how they interact with you*) to determine who you wish to work with. If two doctors recommend the same treatment plan, you'll probably want to choose the doctor who has the *better* bedside manner. The one who asks how you're feeling, or makes you laugh, or listens to you when you ask your scariest questions.

For me, the question became "If I have to go through this uncertain journey, how can I do it as comfortably and gracefully as possible?" This meant choosing the most competent doctors I could find who also *made me feel cared for.* For grace, I decided to do my best to relax into this experience, accept what I could about my future, and *with dignity,* walk into my future, whatever it held.

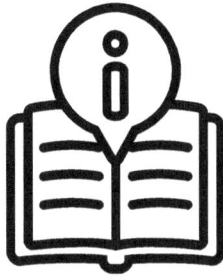

Chapter 04

How to Get the Support You Need

The Cancer Companion

A cancer diagnosis can feel very isolating.

I know it's hard to ask for help, especially if you've spent most of your life taking care of other people. And let me be clear, you can absolutely "do" cancer alone. But it makes something that is *very hard* even *harder.* Harder on you, and harder on the people who love you. Because, you see, a cancer diagnosis doesn't just impact the person diagnosed. It sends shock waves through the circles of people around you; those who care about you and will want to help you through this crisis.

When I received my first diagnosis, I remember feeling as if I was all alone on a deserted island of panic while the rest of the world was busy blissfully going about living their lives. I knew my death was imminent while they seemed oblivious to my mortality, or their own. I felt as if everyone, including my family and friends, was busy partying on the shore, within my view but outside of my reach, while I was miles away on my own private cancer island.

But a number of people sent lifelines to me on cancer island. These came in the form of texts and phone calls and in-person visits. In time, when I could trust myself to keep it together, I was able to gather those friends and family around me for help. Because I needed help.

Sometimes the strongest thing we can do – for our sanity and our survival – is admit to ourselves that asking for help is okay. It can improve our cancer journey and our outcomes. It's hard to think straight when you first hear the diagnosis. I'd like to ask you to consider how you can start to build a group of people you trust to help you deal with the challenges to come. This chapter will offer some easy-to-implement ideas for building your team.

Gather Your Support Network

Consider making the first people you tell those whom you believe could be most helpful to you. These priceless souls will drive you to and from appointments and/or join you in the room with the doctor. You'll treasure having people around who you are most comfortable being vulnerable with because there will be times when you will feel, and be, vulnerable. They could be "framily" – your chosen family. This is your innermost circle of trust and support, your "team." The people you know will show up. No matter what.

Your support network may evolve/expand over time as more people learn of your cancer and want to help in any way they can. It may also evolve as you become more comfortable asking for help.

Consider Keeping Your Health News Private Until You Know more About Your Treatment(s) and Prognosis

This was a painful, but key learning for me when I was diagnosed with cancer. The first weekend after my diagnosis, and before we had spoken with the doctor(s) who would be prescribing and administering my treatments, we *called every member of our immediate family to tell them I had cancer.* Understandably, our family members had questions and we had NO answers for them. All we kept saying is "We don't know, we don't know..."

The impact was horrible. Our families were sad, scared, and stressed upon hearing the news. We took what was a bad situation for us – not knowing what the future might be – and we inflicted it upon every member of our family. Of course, the dizzying number of unanswerable questions they had, coupled with the sad fact that we had no idea what the future held, took its toll on us too.

It does not need to be like this. There is another way.

To be clear, I'm not saying you shouldn't share this initial scary news with a small subset of people. You absolutely will want to share it with your innermost circle. What I am suggesting is that it might be easier on everyone involved if you wait a week or two while you gather the information about your prognosis and your treatment plan, *and then* share your health news more broadly. You'll be better equipped to answer questions. This also gives you time and space to help guide how those who care about you can think about your cancer. (More on that in Chapter Six.)

Do Not Feel Bad if You Don't Invite Everyone into Your Innermost Circle

It is totally acceptable to keep your support network small if you want to be more private. Include the people who will provide the kind of help and encouragement you need. Do not feel obligated to include anyone else. This is a time in your life where *your needs* supersede all others. If you want permission to prioritize yourself above everybody else – you have it. I just gave it to you.

And yes, this is complicated if you are a caregiver for other people (a child, an elderly parent, etc.), but perhaps your support network can help you with those responsibilities. Which brings us to the next topic...

Start a List of Activities Where You Would Welcome Help

When people hear of your cancer diagnosis, many will react by asking "How can I help?" While this is absolutely well intentioned, it can feel absolutely overwhelming to someone with a very long cancer "to do" list. The request for "some way to help" from well-meaning friends can feel like yet-another-task added to an already interminable list of doctors' appointments, scans, and tests. I remember thinking "Gosh. How CAN you help? Can you cure cancer?"

You might feel like you have no idea what you will need. That is understandable. You don't know what you don't know. Not yet.

So...one of the proactive things you can do is start a list of things you would like help with. Then, when someone asks, "How can I help?" you have a list at the ready! To help with this, I have a starter list of suggestions in the appendix of this book. It is not exhaustive; it is simply meant to get you thinking about where you can deploy your support network. Get creative! Maybe it can even become something fun? Maybe?

A close childhood friend of mine told me that once he was diagnosed with cancer, he announced to his husband that he could no longer wash dishes because he had cancer. I'm not sure his husband bought it, but it made them both laugh in a gallows humor kind of way.

And if it really IS overwhelming and hard when someone asks how they can help, consider sharing that fact with them. Maybe say something like "Gosh, I wish I knew, but this is all very new to me and I am still getting my footing. Perhaps you can check in again in a couple of weeks when I have a better idea of what I need? Thank you."

OR assign the "How can I help" questions to someone in your support network. When people ask "How can I help," you can say "Please speak with Geoff, he'll know what needs doing! I am wholly focused on getting rid of this cancer and am finding I can't focus on another thing!"

Talk with Family/Friends/Trusted Co-workers Who Have Had Cancer

If there are people already in your network who have had cancer, you'll likely find it helpful to speak with them about their experience. While what that person went through will not necessarily reflect what you will, sometimes it is just helpful to speak with someone who *knows* you. Because this person is part of your trusted circle, they may be particularly good at listening to your concerns and helping you re-frame them. Or they may have "tips and tricks" for what helped them get through their cancer journey.

However, if people-you-know-who-have-had-cancer fall into the category of unhelpful-people-who-make-you-feel-worse, then absolutely forget this advice and move on. You have no obligation to speak with anyone who makes you feel bad or freaks you out more. What is most important right now is that you take care of yourself – physically, mentally, and emotionally. And if that means avoiding certain people, so be it. Again, I give you permission.

Explore In-person Support Services

Many medical centers offer services such as support groups, yoga, meditation, and nutrition & cooking classes. For many cancer patients, these groups create a safe space for them to speak openly about their hopes and fears with other people going through similar experiences. I think this can be especially helpful if it occasionally feels like the people around you "don't get it" because they haven't had cancer. These gatherings provide you with the opportunity to interact with someone, or more than one someone, who *does get it.*

I found working with a nutritionist to brainstorm what "soft foods" might not hurt my mouth while undergoing radiation treatment (answer: scrambled eggs and chicken broth with truffle salt!) to be super helpful. I found my experience of speaking to a REAL person more helpful, and reassuring (and more empathetic) than googling "soft foods" (answer: smoothies and yogurt, both of which stung in my mouth of cold sores)!

Explore Online Support Services

If your medical center doesn't offer support services (or in-person events don't feel like your thing right now) organizations like the

American Cancer Society (Cancer.org) offer online services. Check out their "programs & services." These often include seriously terrific stuff like free rides to treatments, free lodging during treatment, and a 1-800 number you can call 24 hours a day, 7 days a week if you need it. Even if you don't need it, it's nice to know it's there, right?

Note: Please seek professional help immediately if you are overwhelmed and contemplating self-harm. You're dealing with a LOT right now and talking with someone about it may help you to work through the overwhelm you are feeling.

Work with a Physical Therapist

Cancer treatments, specifically surgery and radiation, can lead to new physical limitations. Doctors can prescribe sessions with a physical therapist to help you gain back strength that was lost and/or devise new ways of adjusting to these limitations. Insurance will often cover the cost of these treatments.

My breast surgeon removed twelve lymph nodes to determine if the cancer had spread to my lymphatic system (result: two of twelve had cancer in them). The lumpectomy combined with the removal of the lymph nodes resulted in me having frozen shoulder. I didn't even know this existed as a side effect before I was no longer able to raise my arm overhead! I went to physical therapy to learn exercises that would help stretch out my shoulder. Eventually I regained full movement of my arm. Huzzah!

Consider Prescribed Medications to Help Ease Your Anxiety and Get Much Needed Rest

When I was diagnosed with two separate cancers within two months of one another, I panicked. I thought about cancer from the moment I woke up until the time I went to bed and tried (and failed) to sleep. I could not stop catastrophizing, anticipating that THE WORST was coming. I began to imagine this panic I was feeling was actually going to result in a heart attack long before either of my cancers could kill me. At my wit's end, I asked my breast oncologist to prescribe an anti-anxiety medication. She did. Every day at 4 p.m. (the witching hour for me when my panic hit the apex) I would take this pill and it would take the edge off. By bedtime, I could fall asleep. I could rest. And once I began to rest, I began to relax.

I wish rest and relaxation for you. I know those might feel far away right now, but medications (and/or meditation/yoga/energy work/

acupuncture, which we will cover in Chapter Ten) may help. What you need right now is sleep and stress reduction so your body can go to work with the doctors and their treatments to get rid of this cancer.

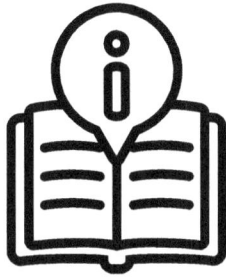

Chapter 05

How to Be Your Own Best Advocate

The Cancer Companion

Everyone who has had cancer (or works in the medical field) will tell you this, but it is important to remember: **you are your own best advocate**. No one will have the same sense of urgency about your health as you will. No one understands as well as you do what is going on in your body: physically, mentally, and emotionally. You are an expert when it comes to YOU. No one is a more compelling advocate when it comes to your health and well-being. Honest.

You may have already experienced this in simply getting to your diagnosis, but there can be weeks and months between doctor appointments. There's the scans and tests you need to do to get a diagnosis, and more waiting time to get a treatment plan. No one will place as much importance on moving this along as you will. It is not that they do not care, but they are humans too and have a lot going on themselves. Best not to take it personally and instead become pleasantly persistent with everyone you meet on this journey. Tell them how crucial it is to you to get things done quickly, and they may just help you out! I know this seems like a big pain in the butt when what you want to do is focus on getting healthy, but this IS how you get healthy, faster. You dig down into your internal resources and start advocating for yourself.

And, of course, on days when it seems like it is just TOO MUCH, give yourself some grace and let yourself just be. You can get back on the self-advocacy horse tomorrow, but do get back on the horse. (Okay, pep talk over.)

Here is some guidance for ways you can be an effective advocate for yourself:

Be Proactive and Persistent in Scheduling Appointments

If the scheduler gives you an appointment that is weeks away, take it, but then patiently and relentlessly call to get rescheduled to an earlier date. Patients cancel appointments *all the time.* You can be first on the waiting list. Befriend the scheduler. Get them to work on your behalf.

Be Willing to Travel for Your Tests and Scans (if you can)

Sometimes your medical center has a number of sites where scans or tests can be done. While the medical center will likely offer you appointments at the site closest to you, it could be a long wait to get a scan or test scheduled if that facility is busy. Often, if you simply ask the scheduler about other medical centers that offer what you need, they will find you an earlier appointment elsewhere. If you are willing to travel (drive, or in some cases, fly), this can move up your treatment timeline.

Before I was diagnosed, when I was told it was going to be six weeks before I could get an MRI at my local medical center, I looked for MRI centers near where I was going to be on a business trip. I booked a date that saved me four weeks of waiting, and worrying, time. Unfortunately, I still was told I had cancer, but I reduced the excruciating not-knowing time period.

Write Down All of Your Questions and Bring Them to Your Doctor Appointment(s)

Write down all of your questions even if you think maybe some are silly or awkward. If those questions are keeping you up at night, they are not silly or awkward. Please be gentle with yourself. It is hard when you're getting a lot of information thrown at you to remember every question you want to ask. By writing a list of your questions you can make the best use of your time with your doctor, and you can minimize your need to email them later for clarification or to make follow up appointments.

I kept an ongoing note on my phone. Every time I would have a question, I would type it in. It was kind of like my grocery list, but for cancer questions. Then, at my next appointment, I would pull out my phone and starting going down my list to get my questions answered.

Take Notes

Better yet, have *someone else* take notes. It is hard to listen AND take notes at the same time, so if you bring someone else, s/he can be taking notes while you speak with the doctor and ask follow up questions. By the way, it is not weird to bring someone with you to your appointment. Medical centers are very used to patients bringing caregivers and other support people to appointments.

AND it is a terrific practice to re-read your notes later to ensure you understood what the doctor was telling you. If you and the note taker interpreted something differently, it is okay to follow up via email with your care team for clarification. In my case, I completely missed that my doctor told me my pee would be orange after I had (doxorubicin – the "red devil") chemotherapy. I was absolutely shocked by the color and came racing out of the restroom to tell my husband, Geoff, who replied, "Yeah. They warned us about that. Don't you remember?!"

Nope!

If You Are Confused, Ask for Clarification

Cancer is confusing. It is probably a new vocabulary for you. AND you are likely totally stressed out right now. It is not unreasonable for you to be having trouble remembering or understanding what is happening in these really challenging circumstances. If you don't understand what the doctors are saying, ask them to repeat it or ask them to explain it using different words. If you don't know why you're having a test done (Why a CT scan? Why a PET scan?), ask your doctors. By the way, Chapter Seven is all about scans and tests (and what they feel like).

Be Embarrassingly Honest with Your Doctors

Doctors can only treat you and help you get better if they understand what is going on with your body. It may seem to YOU that the pain and swelling in your arm is something that should naturally just go away – or it could be that you're showing early signs of lymphedema (a swelling caused by too much lymph fluid collecting in a part of the body). If it is lymphedema, the doctors will have ideas for what you (and they) can do to reduce it.

As embarrassing as it might be, you even need to *tell your doctor* if you are experiencing diarrhea or constipation or fevers. Any of these symptoms could be indications of a larger issue at hand (like an infection). At the very least, bringing up an issue helps doctors offer treatment or medications to reduce your discomfort.

If You Need Something, Ask for It

There is no reason to "tough it out" (pain) or be embarrassed (constipation) or be ashamed (depression). Make sure you are giving your team all of the information they need to be successful in the treatment of ALL of you. Your team can't help you if they don't know what you are experiencing.

I had to speak with my doctors about all of the above at one time or another. Finding ways to alleviate some of the physical and mental pain I was feeling helped make my cancer experience better (or at least, less hard).

Ask a Loved One/Friend to Help as Your Advocate

If you're not comfortable or able to advocate for yourself, perhaps your partner/family member/friend would be willing to take on this role. Maybe think of the person in your life who is "pleasantly persistent" and ask him/her to be your advocate. What you want is someone who can help you (and the doctors' offices) keep appointments and scans/tests organized, on track, and prioritized. Perhaps there is someone you know who is particularly skilled at project management? Or who has been through cancer treatments themselves? Even having another person to talk through the options for care can be super helpful.

Ask if Your Medical Center Has a *Patient Advocate* Service

If there isn't a loved one/friend who can advocate for you and coordinate your care, your medical center or insurance carrier may offer patient advocate services to help you with all of this. A patient advocate is someone who can help coordinate your care, will follow up and coordinate all of your doctors' findings and recommendations.

Please note that it is not disrespectful to your doctor if you ask for a patient advocate. Medical centers have created these positions for a reason. It's because sometimes patients need help in the coordination of their care!

Get Insurance Pre-approvals

Some insurance companies have nurse coordinators who are assigned to patients to help them navigate their medical journey, including their insurance coverage. You might be able to have this person help you get approvals (or better yet, pre-approvals) for your much-needed scans and tests. This allows you to speed up the time between your doctor's request and your test or scan appointments.

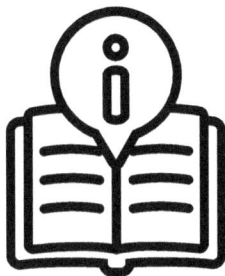

Chapter 06

How to Speak About Your Cancer Diagnosis

Sharing news of your cancer diagnosis can feel awkwardly public about a very private matter (your health). And, because the reactions of the people you're speaking with can be so unpredictable, many of us avoid talking about it altogether. But with some planning and forethought, you can let people know what is happening in a way that feels comfortable for you and on your terms.

Decide How Public You Want to Be About Your Cancer Diagnosis

⋛ **Guidance:** Tell the people you want to tell. Don't tell the people you don't want to tell.

It is your health and you are entitled to keep it as private as you would like it to be. But also understand that once you have told a few people your health news, it may not be realistic to expect that they will keep it private. So, think carefully about who you share your information with as your inner circle of trust might get bigger than you want. People with the best of the intentions may fail to consider your news confidential.

Don't feel bad about *not* telling some people. It is your news. It is your decision whether to tell someone. In the early days especially, when you are still learning about your cancer treatment, you might choose to keep it quiet. As your comfort with the news increases, you might find yourself more open to sharing with more people.

In fact, your opinion on how public you want to be may change over time. That's okay. With my first cancer diagnosis, I wanted to be very private and get through treatment as quickly and quietly as possible. With my second, concurrent diagnosis (and the need for me to take a year off from work for treatments), I decided I would go very public with the news. This included starting a blog. It simply became too tough for me to keep people apprised individually. Both approaches were right for me at the time I made those decisions.

Write Out What You Want to Tell People

Communications experts called these "talking points." Talking points are the messages you want to get across to your audience. They help you stay focused when sharing this difficult news. And in truth, many people will take their cues for how they should react from you. It may also help you to control (or shape) the story others tell about you by allowing you *to tell people how to think about it*. Here are the talking points I created for myself:

I need to share some tough medical news with you.

I have been diagnosed with two forms of cancer.

One really rare cancer that is salivary gland cancer.

And one sadly common cancer that is breast cancer.

The doctors plan to use a treatment plan that will include chemotherapy, surgery, and radiation to ensure they have removed all cancer from my body.

I'm feeling really optimistic because the doctors know how to treat my breast cancer and my prognosis is good.

Consider Starting a Blog or Email Chain to Share Information (updates) Broadly

Once you tell more than about five people about your cancer diagnosis, it may become difficult to remember who you told what to. It can become overwhelming to keep people up to date on your progress and treatments, especially if you have days when you feel lousy.

There are non-profit websites (caringbridge.org is one, lotsahelpinghands.com is another) that allow patients and caregivers to give updates to family and friends during a health crisis. Patients write their updates directly to the site and anyone who has signed up for the blog gets an email alert that an update has been posted. It is important to note that these websites have privacy settings which allow patients to decide how public, or private, they wish to make their updates.

If a blog seems too burdensome, another simple idea might be to write an email to one person and ask that person to forward the email to an agreed upon list of people you wish to update.

Understand People Will Have a Range of Reactions to Your News

Some reactions to your news will be lovely and heart-felt and exactly what you need to hear. ("I am so sorry you're going through this. It must be hard.").

Unfortunately, some other reactions won't always be good or helpful to you ("Oh my God, how long do you have left?" Yep, someone actually asked me this.). Please know that you have no obligation to listen to those unhelpful people and you are not responsible for making them feel better.

One of the challenges in sharing your cancer diagnosis is that people will have a spectrum of reactions, depending on what their prior experience is with cancer. It may have nothing to do with you! Their background will affect how they hear and react to your news. Like you, they may experience any one of the stages of grief, including denial, anger, bargaining, depression and acceptance. Or they may say awkward things because they don't know what to say to you.

AND the reality is that some people may never look at you the same again. You will forever be someone who has cancer and they will associate the disease with how they see you. I still have friends (twelve years after my cancer treatment ended) whose first question when they see me is "How is your health?" It is a well-meaning question but it also tells me that this is now their view of who I am – a cancer sufferer. UGH.

If someone's reaction is not helpful to you, then limit your time with that person until they are able to be supportive and helpful. I give you permission if you need permission. Or maybe lie and tell them that your cancer is contagious so they leave you alone. Again, you are not responsible for making unhelpful people feel better. You are responsible for *you*. That's it. And *that* responsibility is your most important one right now. It's a lot, and it is enough.

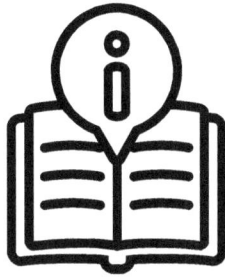

Chapter 07
Scans and Tests

Thankfully (yes, I said thankfully), there are a lot of scans and tests out there that can look for cancer. Unfortunately, they're not perfect. Sometimes they miss stuff (what is called a *false negative*) and sometimes they detect stuff that isn't there (what is called a *false positive*).

In my experience, it is best to schedule ALL tests and scans your doctor recommends. Do every one of them. Get as much information as you can. This way you and your doctors will have a greater picture of your situation and can determine the best course of action. And while sometimes the full picture is not terrific news, at least it is in not the IMAGINED terrible, horrible picture that your brain will catastrophize!

Below are some of the tests and scans that your doctors may recommend. My goal is to tell you what the test is, why it is given, how it feels, and if I have any "guidance" for preparing for it.

Biopsies

Biopsies are taken when doctors want to test samples of a lump to determine if there are abnormal (cancer) cells contained within it.

There are a whole host of different kinds of biopsies doctors might perform, depending on where the suspicious lump is. I'm going to focus on the most common ones.

Needle Biopsy/Fine Needle Aspiration (FNA)

Not surprising, given the name, this biopsy is conducted with a needle that is inserted into the area multiple times to gather enough cells to view under a microscope.

What does an FNA feel like?

To get enough cells to view under a microscope, they need to poke you with the needle ten times. Twice. The experience is kind of like having a sewing machine needle (poke, poke, poke) applied to the area that needs to be biopsied. Some people will have bruising in the area after the procedure. I was given a topical numbing gel for the FNA in my mouth, but I still found the needle pokes painful. It was in my mouth, after all, a very sensitive part of the body. The FNA of the tumor in my breast was less painful.

Excisional/Incisional (Core) Biopsies

There are other kinds of biopsies doctors can order to gather **more** tissue to view under a microscope. An *excisional* biopsy involves the doctor removing the entire lump in order to study it. An *incisional* (or core) biopsy involves just taking a cylindrical sample of the lump in order to study it.

What does a core biopsy feel like?

The instrument used to take the core biopsy kind of looks (and sounds) like a nail gun. (Sound: Thwap! Thwap! Thwap!) A core biopsy extracts more cells (read: more flesh) than an FNA. Doctors use sonograms or MRIs to locate the area they wish to biopsy. In every case where I have had a core biopsy, they have numbed the area first (with a needle full of anesthetic like at the dentist) so it hasn't been too painful.

Sonogram-guided Biopsy

Technicians use a sonogram "wand" that projects images on a screen to locate the area for biopsy. Muscles look like stratus clouds, all stripey and a different shade of gray than the rest of the area. Major veins show as black spots, as do tumors. Once the area for biopsy has been identified, they anesthetize the area and use the (nail gun) instrument to (thwap!) take the biopsy.

MRI-guided Biopsy

The technician injects the area with anesthetic and inserts a marker where s/he believes is the location of possible cancer cells. The doctor then uses a "boring" machine (even more advanced than the nail gun used to do the core biopsy) to bore into the lump and pull out a full gram of tissue to be tested.

MRIs

MRI stands for Magnetic Resonance Imaging. It is basically a scanner machine that has a big magnet in it. You (in a hospital gown with no metal on your body) are conveyor-belted into the MRI machine and a technician uses magnetic fields to take pictures of your body in 2D and 3D. MRIs can capture images of soft tissue and (bonus!) don't use radiation.

What does an MRI feel like?

There is nothing painful about an MRI. It is just freaking loud. And, it is a tight space to be in. The MRI machine looks like a big, plastic white tunnel with a pallet sticking out of it. The pallet is the table you will lie on in order to be conveyor-belted into the machine.

Some MRI scans require that the patient have "contrast" injected intravenously (in your veins) in order to show greater contrast between tissues and body structures. This helps the doctor to see greater definition of a tumor, for instance. If your doctor wants this contrast, it means a nurse will set you up with an IV prior to the scan. During the MRI, the technician will let you know when they're about to inject the contrast. When they inject the contrast, you'll feel coolness in your arm as it makes its way into your bloodstream. It's not painful but the nurse will suggest you drink plenty of water (approximately eight cups) afterward to flush the contrast out of your system.

> **Guidance**: MRIs are big machines that generate a lot of heat so the air conditioning will be on full blast in the room. If you are someone who gets cold, ask for a heated blanket (or four!). MRI technicians have blanket warming machines that are simply magical.

⋛ **Guidance**: The technician will also offer you headphones and/or earplugs. Earplugs are a must. Do **not** go into the MRI without the earplugs. Remember the whole "There is nothing painful about an MRI" comment, above? Well, there IS if you don't wear earplugs – the MRI is *that loud*.

Once you are on the pallet, with earplugs and blankets in place, the technician will hand you a cord with a "panic" button at the end of it. The great news is that if something bad were to happen (which it won't), or if you really do launch into a full-blown panic attack because the space is so small, you can press the button and they'll stop the scan. That's the good news. The bad news is...they'll stop the scan. And you really do want the scan so your medical team can have the best view of what is going on inside your body.

⋛ **Guidance:** Two options exist for you if you just don't think you can do the small space. One option is an "open" MRI machine. It is more open but the imaging isn't as clear as with a "closed" MRI. The other option is to request a general anesthetic during your MRI so that you sleep through the whole experience.

Note: You can't move during an MRI because it makes the scan blurry (think of times you've missed a photo because you moved the camera). However, technicians have microphones to the machine and will speak with you between scans to let you know when you can move and when you must remain as still as a statue.

CT scans

A CT scan (also known as a CAT scan) is a computed tomography scan. It is a scan that uses X-rays to take 3D pictures of the body. The benefit of this scan is the images can be "cut" many different ways to get different (better) angles of the internal organs and tissues of the body. Another great thing is that the machine doesn't require the patient to be conveyor-belted into a long tunnel as it's much shorter and (truly) donut-like in shape. It's a pretty easy and fast procedure. The more controversial part about this kind of scan is the fact that the patient is exposed to radiation during the scan.

What does a CT scan feel like?

For a CT scan, technicians also use a contrast liquid injected intravenously to aid in image creation. Like the MRI, a nurse will give you an IV prior to the beginning of the scan. Then you'll lie down on a table, this time in front of a donut-like machine. The technician will explain how the test will work, and then they'll leave you in the room with the machine. This time, when they inject the contrast, you'll feel a warmth moving through your veins. Then the funniest thing will happen. The warm you feel will begin to concentrate itself in your crotch (!!) and then it's gone. A CT scan is pretty quick, probably twenty minutes total. Once again, the nurse recommends you drink a lot of water afterward to flush out the contrast.

Bone scans

This is a nuclear scanning test to look for abnormalities in the bone – such as fractures or the spread of cancer to the bones. Radioactive (!!) liquid is injected into your veins in advance of the test and then the scanner takes internal pictures of your body by detecting the radioactive materials.

What does a bone scan feel like?

This is not painful at all but is a little freaky (it was to me!) because of the radioactive liquid. You lie on a table with a machine overhead that scans your bones to see if there is evidence of cancer in your bones. It takes thirty to sixty minutes total.

PET scans

A PET scan is a "Positron Emission Tomography" scan. It is also a nuclear imaging scan used to produce a 3D image for doctors to detect cancer metastases (e.g. when cancer has spread to other parts of the body). MRI and CT scans are used to determine what is going on anatomically in the body. PET scan helps doctors to understand what is going on metabolically (what's going on biochemically in the body), so often these are used in conjunction with one another.

What does a PET scan feel like?

This is not a painful test. Like the bone scan, it is a little freaky because the nurse injects you with radioactive liquid prior to the test. It takes about an hour for the radioactive stuff to make it through your system. Then they take you into a room with a big machine with gigantic arms. You lie down on a table and the arms scan over you like some large photocopy machine. You have to lie really still so that the machine can take a picture of your bone structure. This is a super cool picture to look at because you can see your skeletal form. The radioactive stuff goes where there is a lot of "bone turnover" activity – effectively where there is a concentration of rapidly reproducing cells (which is what cancer does). The areas with a lot of activity show up in black on the scan while your bones show up as light grey. It takes about thirty minutes to do this test. And once again, you're going to want to drink water afterward.

Test results

> **Guidance:** Keep copies of all of your test and scan results. This way you can quickly and easily provide copies to doctors you seek for a second opinion, or those you are referred to.

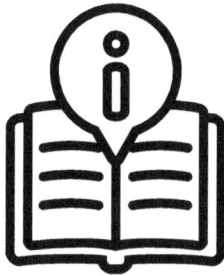

Chapter 08
Surgery

Surgery is a pretty common option, if available, to remove cancer from your body. The surgeon cuts out ("excises" in medical terms) the tumor as well as a perimeter around it. The surgeon's goal in extracting the extra flesh is to try to achieve what are called "clean margins." The doctor includes a larger area around the lump to ensure the area remaining has no cancer cells in it (is "clean").

Once the surgeon has removed the cancer-infected areas, s/he sends it to the lab. They look under a microscope to see if there are any malignancies at the perimeter, which hopefully covers the margin. It is important to note that different medical teams define "clean" by different measurements. Some teams feel they have achieved "clean" margins if there is a clean 1 cm area around the tumor removed, for other teams it is 2 cm, and even as large as 5 cm(!!).

If the surgeon does **not** achieve clean margins (they still see cancer cells in the outer part of the perimeter), you may need to have additional surgeries to remove greater margins until a "clean" margin is achieved. I received a phone call from my surgeon two weeks after my initial surgery to let me know that the radiology team had looked at my excised flesh and detected cancer cells close to the edge. While it was a huge bummer to hear I needed to have another surgery, I also knew I **wanted** the doctors to get it all out, so back to the hospital I went. We achieved clean margins with surgery number two.

What happens during surgery? What does it feel like?

Prior to surgery

Two weeks prior to surgery, your medical team will ask that you stop taking pills like aspirin, fish oil, and Advil (or ibuprofen). All of these supplements thin your blood and impair its ability to clot. During these no-Advil-days, I had to turn to Tylenol, though it just reminds me why I started taking Advil in the first place. Tylenol does little to reduce my pain.

You'll be asked to stop eating eight hours prior to your surgery. This is to ensure you have an empty stomach so you don't have a negative reaction (read: nausea and, likely, vomiting) to the anesthesia they're going to give you. Surgery is tough, but surgery plus vomiting is worse. So don't eat!

Day of surgery

On the day of your surgery, they'll ask you to show up a couple of hours early to prepare. They will tell you not to bring any valuables, but you **will** be asked to bring (and show) your ID. I think this is funny and ridiculous. Who in their right mind is going to impersonate you and **willingly** have a doctor cut them open? But anyway, the hospital wants to make sure they have the right person. Did I forget my ID when I left the house at 4 a.m. on the morning of my first surgery? Of course I did, but they still took me!

Once they have confirmed your identity, you'll be handed a hospital gown to change into. This is a very unfashionable but easy-to-open top with mis-matched pants. Then you'll be told to put all of your clothes into a bag that you will carry with you all day long. This same bag will end up in your hospital room if you're spending the night. I would strongly suggest you bring your own entertainment (A book? A trashy magazine? Your iPad so you can play the New York Times crossword in easy mode?) to distract you while you wait-and-wait-and-wait for your surgery. There may be a television in the waiting room but, honestly, since when is daytime TV interesting?

If you are lucky, you may be placed into a private hospital room. Then you'll be ushered into a waiting "bay." Basically, the surgery bay is a big room with curtains hanging from the ceiling between hospital beds to create the illusion of privacy for all of the folks lying on those beds waiting for their surgeries. A nurse will insert an IV into your arm so they can give you fluids during your surgery. Then you will wait until your surgeon decides s/he's ready for you.

Once everyone is ready, you'll get wheeled into your surgery room. There will be a surprisingly huge room with a seemingly large team of people (five to seven?) waiting there for you, including probably a couple of nurses, medical technicians, an anesthesiologist, and your surgeon. I found they're pretty good about talking you through each step of the procedure as they prepare for surgery (e.g. "Okay now we're going to move you to the operating table...") but you can also ask questions if anything seems weird or you're curious or you're nervous.

When the team is ready to start the surgery, they will put a mask over your face to supply oxygen to you and ask you to count back from ten while the anesthesiologist administers the general anesthetic via your IV. You'll be out faster than you think. My bet is you won't make it to five.

After the surgery

After surgery they will wheel you into a recovery room with other folks who are also waking up from their surgeries. Waking up from anesthesia is kind of like waking up from a SUPER HARD sleep – the kind where it takes you awhile to recognize you're re-entering the world of the living. And you will be SO THIRSTY!! The nurse will offer you ice chips to suck on to help with your thirst. They will seriously be the best ice chips you have ever had.

Depending on how involved your surgery was, you may need to spend a night (or more) at the hospital. This allows the medical team to keep an eye on you while you recover. The good news is the medical team will check on you regularly to ensure your body is healing, you aren't in too much pain, and your body remembers how to go to the bathroom. The bad news is they will check on you in the middle of the night while you're trying to sleep. The other bad news is hospital food, but you can always order food delivery or bring your own in.

Once the team has determined that your recovery is underway and your pain is managed, they will require you to walk the length of the hallway on your own AND they will require you to go to the bathroom as living proof that your body has remembered how to evacuate all of that hospital food.

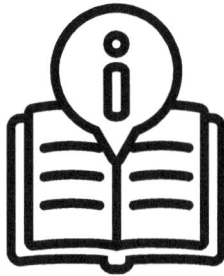

Chapter 09
Radiation

Sometimes surgery is all that is needed to remove cancer from your body. But in other cases, in abundance of caution, the medical team might suggest you do radiation to target any cancer cells that might not have been removed during the surgery. Or, if you are a lucky duck, the medical team might suggest that you *only* need to do radiation (not surgery, not chemotherapy, not immunotherapy, etc.) in order to remove the cancer from your body. Well done, you.

Radiation

Radiation is a targeted therapy doctors use to kill malignant cells. It can be administered before or after surgery and/or chemotherapy, depending on the current standard of care (reminder: this is what your medical team deems the most effective and accepted treatment) for your cancer. Radiation uses "ionizing radiation" (yes, I know I'm not supposed to use the same word to describe a word, bear with me) to kill the cells. Basically, I thought of it as one big laser beam focused on my head (and later, my breast) to "zap" any of the remaining cancer cells still hanging around, post-surgery. Generally, radiation therapy is given every day (except weekends because apparently tumors don't grow on weekends) for thirty-three days.

My understanding is radiation should start about two weeks after surgery to allow the surgery area to heal some, but to still make it soon enough (post-surgery) that the doctors hope to "catch" any errant cancer cells near the surgery site before they move to more distant parts of your body. I have heard of folks requesting their radiation begin farther out than two weeks, for example, when they have a trip already scheduled, but that's not the norm. If you have an extenuating circumstance, I would simply discuss it with your doctors to understand the ramifications of delaying treatment. You will get a vote in your treatments, though I would suggest you follow your doctors' recommendations as best you can.

What does radiation feel like?

I had not given any thought to how radiation would feel prior to the first time I walked into the radiation clinic. I changed into the hospital gown that was handed to me and I was led into a room that had five-foot-thick walls. I lay down on the retractable bed below the radiation machine. Then the technician placed the radiation mask that was created in a prior session on my head. Once I was outfitted in my garish garb (for battle?), the technician left the room by closing that five-foot-thick door and I was ALL ALONE with what looked like a laser beam focused at my head.

I suddenly found myself contemplating what a laser beam blast might feel like (I am a Star Wars fan, so visions of the Death Star blasting the planet Alderaan popped into my head) and I started hyperventilating.

Thankfully, I felt no pain once the technician announced she was beginning the treatment and the laser beam started beeping at me. For about thirty seconds the laser beam moved from one side of my head to the other while I frantically chanted my loving-kindness mantra ("May I be happy. May I be healthy. May I be at peace.") to try to distract myself. The radiation procedure wasn't painful, though the side effects from my head and neck radiation hurt like the dickens (see prior comment about the seventeen cold sores in my mouth!). I had very little pain at all from my breast radiation.

So, let's discuss side effects....

Side effects of Radiation

It bears repeating that every **body** is different, so different bodies have different reactions to radiation. Just because one person experiences a side effect doesn't mean you will. You will find many lists of side effects people have experienced with radiation and chemotherapy. I outline the ones I understand to be most common in this and later chapters, many of which I experienced, however your body may not experience any of them. Wild, huh? (And good news!)

You may have also heard that side effects are "cumulative." In other words, they build up/increase the longer you are irradiated (exposed to radiation). The key is to pay attention to your body as you progress in your treatment. If you have concerns about any of the side effects you are experiencing, speak with the technician or your doctor about them to understand what you can be doing to reduce those side effects.

"Sunburn"/skin changes/soreness

The area being irradiated may become pink and probably painful. Over the counter pain relievers can help. For some folks, the skin might "break down" (get rough and scabby) and you may develop sores, especially at the skin "folds." Again, your doctor may have ideas for salves that can help heal those areas.

> ⸽ **Guidance:** Do not apply lotion to the area being irradiated until *after* the treatment. If you apply beforehand the lotion will intensify the radiation and contribute to skin breakdown. You don't want this. Applying lotion after radiation will help moisturize the area and help keep skin breakdown at bay. That's your goal. I used *Weleda Calendula face cream for babies* religiously and my skin didn't break down.

> ⸽ **Guidance:** Drink lots of water. It is helpful for your skin (and combats skin breakdown) to be as hydrated as you can be. Yes, you will pee more, but it is worth it!

Some folks report permanent "tanning" or changes (firmness) to the skin radiated. I found, and still find, the smooth muscles that were irradiated beneath my jaw and beneath my chest have a tendency to tense up/spasm, but I massage them out and it is fine.

Fatigue

Yes, as radiation therapy progresses (as it accumulates) you might find yourself sleepy in the afternoons.

> ≳ **Guidance:** I instituted a new daily ritual of afternoon napping. And yes, it is still part of my routine. When you find a good thing, don't give it up, I say!

Again, the key is to pay attention to what your body is telling you, and adjust your schedule accordingly, if you can. Remember that the single most important thing you can be doing right now is helping your body be in the best possible shape it can be to tolerate your treatments. If that means napping, by all means NAP!

Hair loss

I didn't experience hair loss associated with radiation, but my radiation was to the jaw and to the breast, neither of which is hairy (for me). My understanding is that this is more common when radiation is being directed at a hairy part of your body (like your head). Significant hair loss becomes more of an issue during chemo (covered in Chapter Eleven).

Mucositis (aka Mouth Sores)

This is inflammation of the mouth or the gastrointestinal tract. Or, as I have described to other people, the WORST FREAKING CANKER SORES OF YOUR FREAKING LIFE. Apparently when you are receiving radiation you are burning 1800 calories/day because radiation:

1. speeds up your metabolism (awesome!) and
2. creates mouth sores (check) *and* you burn calories healing mouth sores?!!

How to deal with (MOFO) mucositis

Stanford Medical Center has this concoction they call "The Stanford Mouthwash" which a very enthusiastic pharmacist tried to tell me was Stanford's equivalent of the University of Florida's Gatorade. (I'm like, "Nope, Gatorade is yummy.") The mouthwash has some combination of numbing stuff and cleansing stuff and the flavor doesn't totally suck (it only sucks slightly). It is meant to numb some of the pain of the mouth sores and help to keep the area clean so it can heal.

> **Guidance:** Keep your mouth as clean as you can and address the pain you have with pain meds (both oral and topical).

Unfortunately, your stomach doesn't really like pain meds (e.g. Morphine, Oxycodone, etc.) when there's no food in it, so you will have to figure out what you can bear to eat. But do remember that the mouth sores *will* heal and you won't die if you can't eat for a couple of days. And truly, with the pain you may not be hungry!

Topical numbing gel can also be a great relief. I applied it pretty regularly during the day to help with the pain.

- **Guidance:** If we were going out, I also would squirt some of the numbing gel into a small snack-sized baggie so that I would have it at the ready if I needed to numb my mouth. I could stick my finger into my jean pocket, and into the baggie, then quickly apply the gel to my mouth sores.

- **Guidance:** Things to eat when you have mouth sores:
    - Ensure (cappuccino is the best flavor, in my opinion)
    - Chicken broth (I highly recommend adding truffle salt)
    - Miso soup with soft tofu
    - Poached eggs, scrambled eggs
    - Cottage cheese

Everyone will suggest milkshakes and yogurt and ice cream to you.

But I found it was best for me to avoid sweet or acidic things as they stung the mouth sores. Also, anything that can break down and get caught in the sores, even cottage cheese, can hurt.

> **Guidance:** One way of getting around the mouth sores is to throw the food to the back of your throat, thus avoiding your swollen mouth. And yes, I'm serious.

The challenge with the whole throw-it-to-the-back-of-your-throat approach is when your tongue also has sores or is swollen, but I found when I needed to eat, using a spoon to throw the food to the back of my throat could lessen the pain and get the food in me.

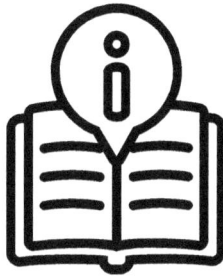

Chapter 10
Pain Management

The Cancer Companion

Unfortunately, cancer can cause pain, whether it is from the cancer itself (a tumor pushing up against an organ) or from surgery (wounds that need healing) or from the side effects of the various treatments (mouth sores from chemo or radiation). The good news is doctors have a whole bunch of medications they can prescribe to you to try to reduce your pain and make it more manageable. Much like nausea, pain is something you want to "stay ahead of" as once you're REALLY EXPERIENCING PAIN, it can be overwhelming.

> **Guidance:** Stay ahead of the pain by following the medication regimen prescribed to you. Sounds really obvious but if you are on top of it, you likely won't have a ton of pain. YAY! But this can trick you. If you stop taking the meds because you think "but I don't have pain" you'll discover without the pharmaceutical help, you WILL have pain.

> **Guidance:** Be honest with your medical team about your pain. Your doctors can't help alleviate discomfort if you don't tell them what you're experiencing. Be clear with them about the frequency and level of the pain you're in.

A note about pain and the overwhelm it can cause: When you're going through intense pain, it can seem like it will never go away. And the thought that you will live with this pain every moment of every day for the rest of your life can be really crushing and hard. Pain medication can help. AND if you can focus on healing whatever it is that is causing the pain, you can get beyond it. There can be a time again without pain. It is important to keep that in mind.

Here's what I didn't know about prescription pain medications, though: the painkillers weren't meant to remove my pain, but only relieve/dull it. UGH. I wanted all soreness gone like when I would have a headache and could pop an Advil to get rid of the headache. Nope. The goal of the prescription pain meds is to relieve moderate-to-severe pain that would be felt on an extended basis (weeks/months/years), but it does not completely remove it. Lame, in my opinion, but here we are.

And you're also only going to know which drug works best for *your body* if you follow the regimen the doctor has prescribed. The first drug or two you try might not work, so you may have to try a couple until you and your doctor find the right balance to provide you relief.

> **Guidance:** Don't be afraid to ask for more pain meds if you have unbearable pain. Your body needs to be able to relax to tolerate your treatment and, ultimately, to heal.

The Cancer Companion

When I first started my treatments, my breast oncologist shared with me that many of her patients were using oxycodone to manage their pain. Having heard how addictive oxycodone can be and well aware of the opioid epidemic in the United States, I told my oncologist that it was my intention to go without pain medications during my treatment as I didn't want to become an addict. She gently suggested that our first order of business was to successfully eradicate the cancer in my body so that I didn't die. If I happened to become addicted to oxycodone, we could deal with that later. It put in sharp relief for me how critical it was for me to be cured of the cancer, a reality that was more urgent than worrying about becoming an addict.

Over the course of my treatments, the pain in my mouth increased to unbearable levels. I was prescribed increasingly stronger pain medications in my desperate search for relief. If, like me, you aren't super familiar with the whole pain medication continuum, let me share with you some of what I learned...

For Mild to Moderate Pain

Nonsteroidal Anti-Inflammatory Drugs (NSAIDs) or Pain Relievers

- **Aspirin** (brand name: Aspirin). This was the first nonsteroidal anti-inflammatory drug (what the doctors refer to as NSAIDs) I was ever introduced to. I take a baby one every day to discourage blood clots (after suffering one in 2006 after a long flight to Ireland).

- **Ibuprofen** (brands: Advil, Motrin, Aleve). This is my go-to drug to fight a headache or body ache. I buy Advil at Costco if that gives you any idea how much I love this NSAID. Apparently, ibuprofen can be tough on the liver, so the doctors ask that you don't use it when you're going through chemo (when your body is already doing a lot of processing in the liver).

- **Acetaminophen** (brand name: Tylenol). Acetaminophen is much easier on the liver than ibuprofen, so this is the drug the doctors encourage you to take while you're undergoing chemo.

Moderate to Severe Pain

Narcotic Pain Relievers

> **Codeine** is a narcotic (opioid) pain reliever. Codeine is often combined with acetaminophen (Tylenol) or aspirin to better relieve pain. You need a prescription for this because, yes, it is addictive. I see codeine as the first line of defense in the war against pain. If that doesn't work, then you move to...

> **Hydrocodone (Zohydro ER)** is a narcotic (opioid) pain reliever. It is often combined with acetaminophen (Tylenol) to reduce pain on a daily, long-term basis. Hydrocodone based brand names include Vicodin, Lorcet, Lortab, Norco, and a whole bunch more. Yes, to needing a prescription, and yes to this drug being addictive.

> **Oxycodone** is a narcotic (opioid) pain reliever that has gained notoriety due to its central part in the current opioid epidemic plaguing the US. Brand names for Oxycodone include Oxycontin, Roxicodone, and Oxecta. Yes, to needing a prescription, and yes to this drug being highly addictive.

⋛ **Percocet** is a combination drug consisting of oxycodone (see above) and acetaminophen (Tylenol). It is meant to reduce moderate-to-severe pain and fever. Yes, to needing a prescription, and yes to this drug being highly addictive.

Breakthrough Pain

Breakthrough pain is "A sudden increase in pain that may occur in patients who already have chronic pain from cancer, arthritis, fibromyalgia, or other conditions" (source: National Cancer Institute). In my case, tantrum and foot-stamping-inducing pain.

⋛ **Morphine** is a chemical found in the opium plant and is a narcotic (opioid) pain reliever. This drug requires a prescription and is highly addictive. I did not love this drug one bit. It made me barf. I wish you better luck with it, but actually, what I am more hopeful for you is you don't have "breakthrough pain."

How do these pain medications work?

For the NSAIDs, the reading I've done indicates doctors are not entirely sure how these pain relievers work. They seem to relieve inflammation that might be the cause of your mild pain. These aren't addictive drugs, so maybe it's okay that we don't know how they work?

For the narcotics/opioids (which are highly addictive), it seems the doctors have a better idea of why they work. "Narcotics work by attaching themselves to pain receptors in your brain. Pain receptors receive chemical signals sent to your brain and help create the sensation of pain. When narcotics attach to pain receptors, the medicine can block the feeling of pain" (source: MedlinePlus.gov). These are terrific things when you are experiencing a lot of pain! The trouble is narcotics/opioids can also create a "high" which many have found addictive. I personally never experienced the high folks speak of, but I wonder if that's because I stopped taking the drugs while I was still experiencing some amount of pain? I don't know.

Side Effects of Pain Medications

While pain medications can do a great deal of good (relief from pain), they can also have pretty significant side effects that you should be aware of. These side effects include constipation (more on that in Chapter Eleven), nausea, vomiting, lightheadedness, headaches; it's a long list, but that's for starters. Pain meds can cause liver damage. They can also "interact badly" with alcohol or other drugs (read: you could die). And, again, some of these narcotics can be highly addictive. Even with all of the "cons" listed against pain medications, I would still encourage you to use them (responsibly and according to your doctor's prescription) to help get you through your treatments.

Cannabis (Marijuana)

Why use Cannabis? It can relax you, ease your pain, reduce your nausea, help you sleep, increase your appetite and a whole range of other reprieves beyond "getting high" that you might seek when undergoing cancer treatments.

At the time of my cancer treatments, cannabis was legal in California only for medicinal purposes. I contemplated applying for a cannabis card to allow me to buy from one of the five dispensaries within a two-block radius of my San Francisco Mission District condo (no joke), but I did not. I don't really have a good answer for why. I have never been a smoker so the idea of smoking to ease the pain in my mouth did not sound appealing whatsoever. But cannabis comes in so many forms now (edibles, oils, drops, etc.) that I imagine I could have found something that worked for me. If I'm honest, I'm kind of bummed out with myself. I should have totally experimented when I had the medicinal excuse and no job to go to!

Cannabis plants produce compounds called cannabinoids; the two most common are cannabidiol (CBD) and tetrahydrocannabinol (THC). THC is the cannabinoid that is so controversial as it's the one that is psychoactive and gets people "high." It's also currently illegal in some states. CBD, on the other hand, is often used for pain relief and inflammation. It's available legally in more states than THC. These cannabinoids can be consumed by smoking, vaping, eating, applying salves or oils, etc. If you want to read more about it, there are websites. For example, www.eaze.com has a whole section for beginners to guide you through the options as well as whether CBD and THC are legal where you live.

My understanding is the TCH products available these days are much more potent/concentrated than they were a decade or so ago, so folks should be careful as they wade into this pain relief option. The key (as with the pain medications I outlined above) is to experiment to find what provides relief for you, but do so carefully. Like pain meds, every *body* is going to absorb/react differently to cannabinoids. Start slow and give yourself time and space to see what works for you.

Drug Disposal

Once I finished undergoing my cancer treatments, I started to think what a target our medicine cabinet would be for a drug addict looking for a fix. Homelessness and addiction were big issues where I lived. Consequently, I decided to take all of my remaining drugs to a local pharmacy where they could properly destroy them rather than:

1. Me selling them to the guy at the end of our street who sits on cardboard all day (kidding) or
2. Flushing them down the drain and into the water supply.
3. **Guidance:** (Eventually) find out where to dispose of unused prescription medications.

In many communities, the police will also receive (and destroy) prescription drugs you no longer need. You can go online to find the pharmacies or police stations in your area that are willing to accept your prescription drugs. My local police station has a mailbox-like bin in the lobby which allows for speedy drop off.

Eastern Practices

Another approach to pain relief is through exploring the mind-body connection of Eastern practices such as meditation, yoga, acupuncture, etc. Prior to my cancer diagnosis I would have told you that I didn't have time for things like yoga and meditation. I had things to DO! I didn't have time to "waste" sitting silently on the floor.

Cancer changed that.

One of the first people I told I had cancer was my dear friend, Tripti. Tripti and I met when we were both working for a financial services company. While I left that company to go to business school and become better at PowerPoint, Tripti left to go to culinary school and later, to a yoga and meditation study program to become a yogi. When I told Tripti that I had cancer she said to me, "I am so glad to hear you'll be getting treatment at Stanford for this cancer. Let's call them Team One—they're your Western medicine team. I'd like to be in charge of Team Two—your Eastern medicine team. Will you let me do that?"

My gateway practice was one called Guided Imagery (which I spoke about in Chapter Two). Once I experienced the benefit of the mental escape provided by Guided Imagery, I became more open to exploring the other practices Tripti recommended. I began taking Tripti's yoga classes multiple times a week. I started meditating. I took advantage of the Healing Touch energy work offered (for free!) at Stanford Medical Center where I was being treated. I indulged in weekly acupuncture sessions (again, someone Tripti introduced me to). I found these practices calmed me. Grounded me. Allowed me to slow down and be fully present for the amazing life I had and was trying to save through aggressive cancer treatment.

While my Western medicine team (team one) saved my body, the Eastern medicine team (team two) saved my soul.

I am by no means an expert in *any* of these practices. I am an enthusiastic beginner so the best I can do is share my highest level of understanding of them. I would suggest if any of these feels compelling, you seek out resources that go into greater detail by people who have dedicated their lives to these practices.

Meditation

This is typically the whole sitting quietly on the floor thing, but it can also be done while moving. The goal of meditation is to focus your mind (and body) to achieve a state of calm and awareness. And it is REALLY hard! But the benefits of it can manifest in a reduction of stress, improved sleeping, and, for me, greater overall calm.

> **Guidance:** Meditation is hard. Your mind wanders. Go chase it and bring it back.

Something I also learned about from Tripti was a practice called the Loving-Kindness meditation. In this practice you might whisper or chant "May I be happy. May I be healthy. May I be at peace." This is a loving plea to the Universe for these beautiful things. Once you have established this "forcefield" (my words) of loving-kindness for yourself, you can extend the chant out to other people whom you know need this love. For instance, while I was going through cancer treatments, my father was also going through cancer treatments, so I would often chant on his behalf. And finally, once you have established that loving-kindness to another person/people, you can extend the loving-kindness to all beings in the Universe.

⋗ **Guidance:** The loving-kindness meditation is a terrific chant to do while getting radiation as it helps you focus on relaxing rather than focusing on the laser beam pointed at you.

Yoga

Yoga is an ancient practice that seeks to bring the mind and body into harmony through physical postures, breathing, and meditation. There are a ton of different types of yoga so it may take a couple of times to find a flavor that you enjoy. I personally love Vinyasa yoga, which focuses on "flow" and coordinating your breath and your movements.

⋗ **Guidance:** Take to heart the fact that yoga is a practice. You will never be, nor are you expected to be, an expert. You are always, simply practicing.

Guided Imagery

As I've mentioned, Guided Imagery was my "gateway" practice. It is now the first thing I recommend to people when they are diagnosed. I start the conversation just as my fertility doctor who first recommended it to me did. "I don't know if you buy into the whole mind-body connection, but for me, the toughest part of cancer was the emotional toll it took on me. What absolutely made it bearable for me was Guided Imagery."

I often describe it to people as meditation but with a guide. And I have no idea WHY it works, but boy did it work for me. I am hopeful it will for you as well. I feel I covered it pretty well in Chapter Two so I'll skip repeating myself here.

Energy Work

Healing touch is a research-based therapy that uses gentle hand techniques by trained practitioners. It provides relaxation and stress reduction to manage the side effects of chemotherapy and radiation treatments.

Healing Touch is an energy-based healing. The practitioner/healer will tailor it to the needs of the individual but the work can be applied while lying fully clothed on a massage table or in a chair.

The practitioner focuses on the seven "chakras" (energy sources) of the body (and yes, the definitions below are over-simplified):

- **Root Chakra** (Muladhara) - located at the base of the spine and representing the foundation of life.
- **Sacral Chakra** (Svadhishthana) - located above the sex organs and is the physical, pleasure-seeking chakra.
- **Solar Plexus Chakra** (Manipura): located at the belly and is the action-oriented (doer) chakra.
- **Heart Chakra** (Anahata): located at the heart. This is the midway point between the lower (physical) chakras and the upper (enlightenment) chakras; it is also the go-between the two.
- **Throat Chakra** (Vishuddha): located at the base of the throat. This is the "power" chakra.
- **Third Eye Chakra** (Ajna): located at the forehead as the center for intellectual enlightenment.
- **Crown Chakra** (Sahasrara): located at the top of the head, believed to be where spiritual enlightenment is located.

I did energy work with a wonderful woman named Sheila who said to me in the first session we had, "Hmmm. You seem to be constipated."

Me: "Um. Yeah. How did you know that?"

Sheila: "I can feel it in your root chakra."

(Me, in my head: "Whaaaat?! What kind of black magic is this?")

Me, out loud: "Huh. What else is my energy telling you?"

Sheila: "You have a blockage in your crown chakra. It seems like you might be mad at God."

Me, in small voice: "Yeah. It's been a challenging time."

Acupuncture

Acupuncture is a traditional Chinese Medicine (TCM) practice where tiny needles are inserted into various parts of the body to release or rebalance the "qi" (energy) of the body. The qi flows through the body via a network of pathways called "meridians." There are twelve primary meridians throughout the body, divided into the "yin" and the "yang" groups.

I had tried acupuncture when I was undergoing fertility treatments prior to my cancer diagnosis. I found the needles super painful; they stung and I couldn't relax. After my first cancer surgery (removing the salivary gland tumor from under my tongue), Tripti suggested I try acupuncture again; this time with her friend Lisa. Hesitantly, I agreed.

Acupuncture hadn't worked for my fertility (I didn't get pregnant) so why would it work now?

Lisa inserted the needles into my body. There was no pain. No stinging. I mentioned this to Lisa.

"You know the fertility meridian ends on the left side of the floor of your mouth, right? Just under your tongue?"

Wait. Where I had had the salivary gland tumor? Was the tumor already there when I was trying to get pregnant? Was the tumor blocking my fertility? *And* was the fertility acupuncture painful because I had a tumor at the end of my fertility meridian? Who knows – but weird.

The acupuncture I did for my cancer treatments was not painful. It was easy and relaxing and a wonderful experience to look forward to after a cancer treatment. And, skeptic that I was, dare I say *healing*?

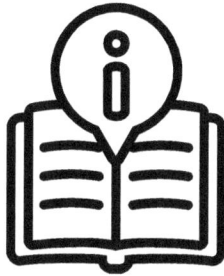

Chapter 11
Chemotherapy

I feel a need to insert a call out to all of those brave people who have gone before us in the cancer journey. Because of their willingness to try out new treatments, doctors have many more effective tools at the ready. Thank you, amazing cancer pioneers.

Among the many amazing therapies currently available, there are over a hundred different chemotherapy medicines, each tailored to be most effective for the cancer it targets. But what is chemotherapy?

Chemotherapy

Chemotherapy is medicine that is administered to kill rapidly reproducing cancer cells. It can be given intravenously (through the veins) or orally (by mouth), depending on the medicine and the standard of care (again, what the most successful treatment for your cancer currently is). It is a systemic therapy, meaning it looks to send medicine to the whole system (your whole body) to kill the cancer cells. My oncologist described it to me this way: "Chemotherapy erases the footprints that cancer may have left in various parts of the body." I really like that image a lot.

How to mentally prepare for chemotherapy

Before I was diagnosed with cancer, I would have told you that chemo is a poison. And I wasn't wrong. Chemo is given to patients to kill their cancer cells. But thinking of it in terms of a poison made me scared and anxious. As I prepared for my first chemo infusion, I decided to reframe how I thought about chemo. I decided to start thinking of chemo as a medicine – something created to heal me from my cancer. For me, this was an important mental shift in how I thought about chemotherapy. It made chemo less scary.

I also decided that my days at the infusion center, while not fun, did not have to be boring and sad. I drove with a different friend or family member to each infusion. I thought of them as my partner-in-crime for the day. Dressing up in cute outfits made me feel beautiful and hip. I brought books to read. My computer accompanied me to tap on. I chatted with my partner-in-crime. Other patients served up interesting conversations too. By intentionally finding ways to keep myself amused, I successfully got through six months of bi-weekly chemo sessions.

⋛ **Guidance:** Invite family and friends to drive you to/from chemotherapy sessions. It is less lonely and more fun.

⋛ **Guidance:** Bring things you enjoy doing (or that will distract you) to every appointment or treatment session you have. There will be delays and time with nothing to do. Entertain yourself.

How to physically prepare for chemotherapy

Pay attention to your body

Most of this chapter is dedicated to discussing the side effects associated with chemotherapy. Some of the side effects might not seem like a big deal, but sometimes a small deal can become a larger problem. Let your medical team know if there are any changes to the way your body is acting as it could be the result of the chemo. If the team has a way of reducing the symptoms, they will do so.

Take special care of your body

Your body has work to do to get this cancer out of you. Now is the time to ensure it is getting the rest (sleep and relaxation), nutrition, water, and exercise it needs to be its most healthy and strong. I am sure you know this intuitively. But if you need someone to tell you, I am telling you. Be kind and good to your body.

- **Guidance:** Get at least eight hours of sleep. Supplement with naps!
- **Guidance:** Eat real food. Don't eat processed food.
- **Guidance:** Drink water! This will help with ALL things.
- **Guidance:** Try to get your body moving every day. It can be a walk. It can be stretching. Just move.

Okay, let's dive into the nitty gritty of chemotherapy.

Delivery mechanisms

Below are the various ways chemotherapy can be delivered to your body.

Intravenous (IVs)

You can choose to have the nurse deliver your chemo via an IV needle to a major vein in your arm each time if you wish. But that can be pretty tough on you and taxing on your veins. If you're going to have regular chemo infusions, you can opt to have the doctor insert a PICC line or a port so that your veins can be accessed more easily, both for you and for medical practitioners. What's a PICC and what's a port, you ask?

(Venous Access) Ports

A venous access port is this totally *rad* device that can be implanted in your chest, arm, or belly prior to beginning treatments. Why in God's name would you do this? Well, if you have small veins or will be receiving regular treatments where the medical folks need to inject stuff into you, the port makes it easier for everyone. The port basically hooks up to the veins and allows nurses and doctors to access your veins simply by "plugging in" to the port. I am pretty sure this is not the medical term for port access, but the port is like this button under your skin where needles can be inserted relatively painlessly (certainly less than so than an IV) and have immediate access to the blood flow. Since my oncologist told me that my chemo would be six+ months of bi-weekly treatments, it made sense to me to have a port installed. Honestly, I thought my port was one of the coolest things I learned about during my cancer treatments. I had thought I would have to have an IV inserted every other week for multiple months like a heroin addict, with similar bruising and damage potential. Not so! I had NO pain or bruising or damage beyond a small scar where the port was inserted. When my chemo was finished and I was preparing for my breast surgery, my oncologist approved my port being removed during the breast surgery. AWESOME.

The only drawback with a port is that it needs to be "flushed" regularly (with heparin, followed by saline) to ensure that it is still flowing into the veins. This is no big deal if you are getting your blood taken regularly (weekly) to "monitor your numbers" or are getting regular chemo. The nurse will flush your port as a part of the overall treatment process. When it becomes a bummer is if you aren't regularly visiting the blood center (maybe you are waiting between treatments) and need to make a special trip there to have your port flushed. Ports have to be flushed at least monthly to remain viable, but this shouldn't keep you from exploring the port option. If it wasn't clear from what I've written above, I'm a big fan of the port and found it helped make my chemo infusions less of a big deal physically.

PICC (peripherally inserted central catheter) line

Less *rad* than the port (in my opinion, though still a viable option) is a PICC line, which is like a semi-permanently set up IV. It is set up via a soft tube with a long soft needle inserted into the veins to allow ongoing access. The drawback here is that to remain viable as an infusion point, PICC lines need to be flushed regularly like ports. But the advantage here is you don't have to have the minor surgery required to have a port inserted into you.

Oral (by mouth)

Depending on the kind of cancer you have, oral chemotherapy might be an option for you. Oral chemo is ingested by the mouth and can be given via tablets, capsules, or liquid. The great part about this is you don't need to go into the infusion center each time you receive this chemotherapy.

Now that we've established how chemotherapy can be delivered, let's talk about the experience of chemotherapy.

What does chemotherapy feel like?

The first chemotherapy session is, of course, the most nerve wracking, simply because you don't know what to expect. As it turned out for me (and for most people), it was not a big deal. I was asked to go to the lab an hour or so prior to chemo so they could take some blood and "check my counts." By "checking your counts," the doctors are checking your red blood cell count, white blood cell count, hemoglobin, hematocrit, etc. They are comparing your counts against the "normal" range of blood counts. If they see any numbers that are "out of range" (low or high) they may choose to have you skip chemo for a week, with the goal of your blood counts rebounding (improving) during the week off.

If your blood counts are in range, your doctor will approve you for intravenous chemotherapy and you will check into the infusion center. Each patient is assigned to a nurse who will administer the chemo and stays watching you to make sure you don't have any adverse reactions. The nurse will start by confirming **who** you are. (Again, WHO in their right mind would impersonate you and go through chemo for you? I don't know.) Once confirmed, they will order your specific medicine from the pharmacy. In my experience it took about twenty to thirty minutes for the medicine to be mixed. During that time, the nurse would set up my infusion site (in my case, via my port) and would start priming me with medicine to help proactively counterbalance any adverse effects I might have from the chemo. Typically, they would give me anti-nausea (there are many different kinds) and anti-inflammatory medications in my IV drip, both of which can help reduce the side effects.

Once finished with these drips (or pills, some come in pill form), they will confirm your identity again and hook you up to your IV bag of chemotherapy. With your first infusion, the nurse will "titrate" the infusion, meaning s/he will give it to you REALLY SLOWLY so they can watch to see if you have an allergic reaction to the medication. I thought this was a GREAT idea because having your first chemotherapy session is kind of like cliff diving. You feel like you are standing at the precipice of a huge drop and you're just not sure if you want to jump or not, but you know you NEED to jump to make yourself better. So, the idea that there is someone there to watch you like an athlete's spotter as you jump, and magically pull you out if it looks like it isn't going well, is just super reassuring. For the three hours that it took for my body to absorb all of the chemo, the nurse was checking in with me every fifteen to twenty minutes to make sure I was still feeling okay. I was also given a panic button (more commonly known as a "call button") that I could press at any time if I started feeling itchy, ill, whatever. All of that made me feel like I had a super big net below me while I cliff dived into chemo.

As far as the infusion itself, I didn't really feel anything remarkable. It wasn't cold. It wasn't hot. It just flowed into me via my port. And when the infusion bag was empty and all of the medicine had gone into my body to begin killing cancer cells, I was excused to go home. Physically, I didn't feel dizzy or in any way weird leaving the clinic, even though mentally I kept thinking "Wow, I have chemo in me. Wow." And I found myself kind of standing outside of myself for the next couple of days, observing and "listening" to all parts of my body to see if any part was screaming out or distressed in any way. Miraculously enough, my body was pretty quiet.

Side effects of chemotherapy

As we've discussed, every *body* is different, so you just don't know how YOUR body will react to the chemotherapy. The tough part is waiting to see which of the infamous side effects will be visited upon your body. Almost any article or book on cancer will detail a list of potential side effects, but you may (or may not) experience any or all of them.

> ⋛ **Guidance:** Check out what classes your medical center offers you to get as much information available prior to starting your treatments.

For instance, I was handed a "potential infusion reactions" guide that listed symptoms of a reaction:

Mild reaction

- ⋛ Itchy skin
- ⋛ Flushing (redness)
- ⋛ Fever above 100°F
- ⋛ Abdominal cramping, nausea
- ⋛ Achy muscles and/or joints
- ⋛ Pain at the tumor site

Moderate to severe reaction

- ⋛ Difficulty breathing
- ⋛ Chest pain
- ⋛ Feeling lightheaded
- ⋛ Very slow or very fast heartbeat

Not a very encouraging list, I know, but again, you might not experience any of these AND it is helpful to know what to look out for, right? The medical team will give you some medications prior to starting your chemo to anticipate and reduce potential side effects (like headache or nausea). And if you experience any of the above after your chemo infusion, by all means TELL YOUR MEDICAL TEAM! They can prescribe other medications to help reduce or eliminate your distress.

Let's dive into some of the listed side effects:

Mild reactions

Itchy skin

Some folks report an overall body itchiness when they are receiving chemotherapy. It is definitely one of those things you want to report to the attending nurse during chemo if you start feeling itchy, as it can be an indication of an allergic reaction to the chemo. My understanding is that if you're someone prone to allergic reactions, then, bad luck, you may experience similar responses to chemo. Antihistamines such as Benadryl®, epinephrine, and hydrocortisone can help combat this itchiness. I believe these were some of the medications they put into my IV drip prior to the chemo being delivered to me, and in my case, they really worked!

Flushing (redness)

Chemotherapy can impact the blood vessels, causing them to expand and constrict, which leads to the skin having a redness or "flush" appearance. It is generally a temporary thing, but you should let the medical team know if it continues. This was the biggest side effect I had from the first chemo (Taxol) I was given. I woke up the morning after my first infusion and it looked like I had a sunburn (no pain, just REALLY pink skin).

Fever

Chemotherapy can impact your white blood cells; the cells that fight infection. If you have a fever during or after chemotherapy, you should tell your medical team immediately as this can indicate an infection. If your immune system (your white blood cells) is compromised, this can quickly become an emergency. You want to stay on top of this. For instance, my dad had a fever after his first chemo. When my parents mentioned the fever in passing to me, I told them to get to urgent care quickly as he might have an infection. He DID. My parents didn't connect that the fever might be related to his cancer treatment. Had he not gone to Urgent Care, his infection could have progressed to something life threatening. I can understand how easily stuff like that happens because you want life to be *normal* when you are going through cancer treatment, but you also have to be vigilant and keep close tabs on what's going on with your body.

Abdominal cramping, nausea

Chemotherapy's job is to kill rapidly reproducing cells. Sometimes healthy cells get caught in the crossfire. My understanding is that nausea and abdominal cramping are the result of gastrointestinal cells being killed in the process of killing the cancer cells. But fortunately, oncology teams have all kinds of other drugs they can give you to counter the nausea and other side effects, which is TREMENDOUS.

I think nausea is the most common side effect of chemo. For me, the nausea was kind of like a hangover that lasted for a couple of days. As I liked to joke, I was lucky my life before cancer had prepared me for the hangover of chemo. I knew well the headache, lack of appetite, and general malaise of a hangover so I knew I could power through it. I combatted it with the anti-nausea medications the doctors had prescribed, Advil, lots of water, and sleep.

⋟ **Guidance:** If you can, block out a couple of "lay low" days after your first chemo infusion just in case you feel lousy. Maybe it's a good practice to block out a couple of days after each chemo infusion, just in case. If you feel fine, I give you permission to take a mini-vacation from life as it is these days.

⋟ **Guidance:** Take the pain and nausea medications they give you according to the schedule outlined. Like pain medication, nausea medication is one of those things you want to "stay ahead of" because once the nausea has kicked in, it has kicked in and getting it to go away is harder than preventing it in the first place.

⋟ **Guidance:** If the meds they give you aren't working for the pain or nausea, ask for more or different meds. You should not feel the need to suffer through.

Achy muscles and/or joint pain

Chemotherapy can damage the nerves that send signals to your muscles and joints, resulting in a side effect called neuropathy.

Neuropathy is tingling or numbness or pain in your extremities (fingers, hands, arms, toes, legs) that appears during or after chemotherapy. Something like 75% of all chemotherapy patients experience some level of neuropathy during chemo. Unfortunately, many continue to experience it after chemotherapy is finished because of the damage done to their nerves. The good news is that there are medications that can be prescribed to help alleviate the symptoms, such as gabapentin and cannabis, but it is still challenging for those suffering from it. I notice the joint pain most when I haven't been moving (when I first wake up and try to walk, or have been sitting for a while).

> ⦚ **Guidance:** I find that once I get moving, the pain lessens. But if the pain doesn't decrease, a heating pad, a warm bath or a hot tub can help.

Pain at the tumor site

Chemotherapy's job is to kill cancer cells. If you feel pain at the tumor site, this is likely chemo doing its job and irritating the nerves and tissue around the tumor site. I like to think of this as a good indication that the chemo is working!

⋛ **Guidance:** Like with joint and muscle pain, a heating pad or warm bath can help.

Moderate to severe reactions

Difficulty breathing

Difficulty breathing can be driven by a number of reasons including the chemotherapy irritating the lungs, fluid building up in the lungs, anemia, and inflammation of the airways. These are all legitimate physical effects from the chemo. Difficulty breathing can also be driven by stress and anxiety associated with the chemo infusion, impacting the body's ability to deliver oxygen to the lungs.

⋛ **Guidance:** Alert your medical team immediately just to be on the safe side. Breathing is kind of important for living.

Chest pain

Chemotherapy can damage the heart muscles. This can lead to spasms of the heart (which restrict blood flow and thus decrease oxygen to the heart). These are painful. After I completed chemotherapy,

I was assigned to a cardiologist who administered multiple EKGs (electrocardiogram: a test that monitors the heart's electricity and can help identify whether there is a problem) over a number of years to determine if I had heart damage. I did not.

Woot! Woot!

> **Guidance:** Alert your medical team immediately just to be on the safe side. Chest pain isn't something you want to fool around with.

Feeling lightheaded

Chemo can reduce the number of red blood cells in your body, which can result in anemia. Anemia can lead to lightheadedness as your body may not be receiving enough oxygen in the blood. Dehydration, from not drinking enough water or perhaps from vomiting due to nausea, can also add to the dizziness factor.

> **Guidance:** Keep hydrated! Take your anti-nausea pills! Alert your medical team immediately just to be on the safe side.

Very slow or very fast heartbeat

Again, chemotherapy can damage the heart muscle and lead to irregular heartbeats (arrhythmia), which can result in a very slow heartbeat (bradycardia) or a very fast heartbeat (tachycardia). Either way, tell your medical team if you are experiencing this.

> ⋑ **Guidance:** Deep breaths (or meditation) can help to slow a rapid heartbeat, though alert your medical team immediately just to be on the safe side.

Bonus side effects

And as if the list above wasn't enough, people report other side effects that I thought I'd list out for you, just so you can be on the lookout for them:

General dryness/headaches

Chemotherapy dries you out. I'm not sure why that is. But I found I had low-grade headaches as a result of infusions. I combatted this with lots and lots of water. Water and general hydration are good for you no matter what the ailment. This was definitely true with the chemo.

<Cough> Other areas of your body can also become "dry" and you may want to consider using lubricants if you are sexually active.

My nails became brittle and more cracked than usual. I combatted this with regular mani-pedis (M-Ps). I had actually been told that you should be really careful about having M-Ps if your white blood cell count is low because that makes it harder for your body to combat infection. Thankfully, my white blood cell count didn't go outside of range during my treatments, so I treated myself to periodic M-Ps to keep my nails in shape, and frankly, to spoil myself.

I also developed dark marks on my nails that appeared as a stripe from the nail bed to my finger tip. I hadn't heard this was a side effect so I was pretty surprised when suddenly I had these bizarre stripes, but my nurse confirmed it was the chemo that was driving it. I also heard from other women with breast cancer who told me their nails detached from the nail bed due to chemo. I am told the nails grow back but WHAT A BUMMER.

Chemo brain/brain jumping around/fogginess

You may have heard the term "chemo-brain" used to describe brain function not only during the course of chemotherapy treatments, but also beyond. The most common issues I have heard, and experienced, include trouble concentrating and trouble remembering things. Though, honestly, I'm not sure at this point whether it's the chemo or my age that is impacting my ability to remember why I walked into a room or what was on my only-three-items grocery list. I did some research on WHY we get chemo brain and this is one of those areas where the doctors aren't entirely sure (they call it "practicing medicine" for a reason). Chemo kills fast growing cells, so maybe that's it? Or maybe we're just more tired after chemo. Feeling "foggy" is a pretty common complaint. While I was a list-maker before chemo, I am now obsessed with keeping lists on my phone, on my computer, on any notepad nearby, so I don't forget things.

- ⋛ **Guidance:** Apparently doing crossword puzzles, or any kind of puzzle or game, is great for maintaining your mental agility.
- ⋛ **Guidance:** Exercising regularly is also a great way to keep you alert and healthy. It's both good for the brain and the body.

Hot flashes

I've had more of these post-chemo, due to the hormonal therapy I'm taking (AND more likely because I am in my fifties), but hot flashes can also occur while you're undergoing chemotherapy. Hot flashes are driven by chemotherapy disrupting the hormones in your body. Estrogen is the hormone in charge of regulating body temperatures, so when it is out of whack, you can get a flash of heat leading to unbearable heat and sweat. Yuck.

> **Guidance:** Consider wearing tank tops and/or cotton shirts that are breathable under cardigans or jackets that can be easily removed to allow your body to cool down. Layers rock during and after chemo, in my strong opinion.

Diarrhea (Yup. We're going there.)

Chemo kills fast growing cells, which means cancer cells, but unfortunately, your stomach lining has fast growing cells too. Treatments can impact and irritate your digestive tract, leading to diarrhea. I experienced a lot to this early on in my chemo treatment.

> **Guidance:** Follow the BRAT diet (bananas, rice, applesauce, and toast) if you can eat.

Thankfully, the diarrhea didn't last long for me because I quickly developed constipation.

Constipation (This is the ying to diarrhea's yang.)

Boy, howdy. Turns out, pain medications and anti-nausea medications can cause constipation. And not that "wow-I've-been-travelling-and-my-body-is-a-little-out-of-cycle" casual kind of constipation. Nope. It is the kind of constipation where you think, "Hmmm. Has my poop fossilized? Do I now have some version of a poop plug in my colon that is expanding as it is hardening...and there is no way in hell my butt is going to be able to dilate to the size needed to pass that fossilized plug?!?" Yes. I just said all of that.

I know there are those folks who are daily poopers with a whole ritual about when and where it happens. They can set a clock by their poop. I'm not one of those people. With chemo and pain medications, everything came to a screeching halt. And I noticed that my body didn't seem to think anything was going to happen for quite some time. And my normal standbys: water, coffee, fruit, and vegetables, weren't going to help. I couldn't drink coffee because, with chemo, the smell of coffee had become one of those scents I couldn't stand. I couldn't eat fruit or vegetables due to the mouth sores from my radiation and chemo (acids and sweets hurt more than almost anything else). I tried increasing my water (result: I peed more).

⋛ **Guidance:** Water. Coffee. Fruit. Fiber. Pro-biotics. Stool softeners. Laxatives. Enema. Exercise. ANYTHING that works.

Weight gain/weight Loss

Okay, back to safer subjects...kind of. You know how during times of stress some people gain weight while others lose? Yeah – so cancer fighting is a pretty stressful time. Add to it that you may have nausea associated with your treatments that makes you lose your appetite and lose weight. Conversely, you might be given steroids that cause you to retain water and gain weight. Cancer treatment can be an intense time of weight fluctuations.

I tried to exercise as much as I could during my cancer treatment. My reasoning here was that the stronger my body was, the better it would be able to process whatever treatment I was being asked to endure to fight my cancers. That said, if you are nauseated or in extreme pain, it is super tough to motivate yourself to start bouncing around on a run or in an exercise class.

⋛ **Guidance:** Go easy on yourself regarding your weight. You've got a lot going on. Understand that you might gain weight, you might lose weight. The important thing is that you're fighting as best you can. You can deal with losing or gaining weight back after the treatments are through.

Thrush

The immune system can become compromised during chemotherapy and put folks at higher risk for the development of oral thrush. The symptoms are white lesions in your mouth (tongue/cheeks/roof of mouth), redness and burning, difficulty eating and swallowing, and loss of taste. All of that sounds awful and actually not unlike the mucositis (mouth sores) that I had from the chemo/radiation combination.

> **Guidance:** Brush your teeth and rinse your mouth (maybe with something like Biotene®) to prevent thrush. If you do develop it, your doctors can prescribe antibiotics to treat it.

Loss of taste

Chemotherapy can damage taste buds and other cells in the mouth, making food and drink taste different. Many patients lose interest in eating or drinking because the taste of things can change.

I did not lose my sense of taste with the first chemotherapy I was given (Taxol), and most certainly didn't lose my hankering for my evening glass (or two) of wine. I asked my doctor about that. She shared that the reason doctors advise patients not to drink during chemo is because the liver is already working so hard to process the chemo. Adding alcohol taxes your liver more. I asked if it was therefore okay if I continued to drink a glass of wine a night as long as my liver function continued to look good during my weekly blood tests. My doctor's answer: Yes.

Hot damn! I could still drink wine.

Microdermabrasion aka best facial of your life

I cannot tell you how many of my friends started commenting on how GREAT my skin looked after I started chemo. At first, I thought they were just searching around for nice things to say to me while actively avoiding discussing how BALD I was. But no, in fact, they were just struck by how much my skin seemed to be "glowing." I asked my dermatologist about it, who explained that in the course of chemotherapy killing cancer cells, it actually kills many facial cells. The result is like a whole series of chemical peels or microdermabrasions to your face, giving you this great glow. *How cool is that?* Saved me all kinds of money on facials.

Hair loss

If your cancer treatment involves chemotherapy, you are probably going to lose your hair for some period of time. Again, this has a lot to do with chemo targeting fast growing (cancer) cells. Hair cells are also fast-growing cells, so they get killed too. I think this is a much bigger deal for women than for men as we are societally used to men shaving their heads as they age. Men also naturally experience hair thinning and male-pattern baldness. It is less common for women and therefore when you are a bald woman, you stand out. And the logical quick conclusion others make is you are bald because you are undergoing cancer treatments.

> **Guidance:** Get a short haircut prior to hair loss so you can get used to short hair. You will also have less hair to clean up when it starts falling out. And/or get your hair cut similar to a wig you like so you can acclimate to that hairstyle. It is less jarring when you start to wear the wig as you are already used to that "look."

Bald-concealing options: hats/scarves/wigs

Hats

I found baseball caps to be the best option for me. I already owned a ton of them and believed people didn't register me being bald when I wore a baseball cap. They just saw the cap and moved on.

I bought a really large, floppy hat for days when I needed more of my skin to be covered but I found that I didn't wear it as often as the baseball caps because it felt more formal than I am.

> **Guidance:** Soft fleece or woolen hats that you can wear to bed at night are amazing. Bald is beautiful, but it can also be cold, so having a hat you can sleep in which keeps your head warm in bed is a must. Something like 10% of our heat is lost through our heads. So cover up!

Scarves

I am not a big scarf person. I want to be a big scarf person as I have a number of very cool girlfriends who wear them (yes, they're European). These friends have an effortless stylishness that I aspire to, but I honestly just never remember to accessorize with scarves. Yes, I think a typically preppy woman like me wearing a headscarf screams "CANCER!" but scarves had some very real value in my wardrobe.

> ⋛ **Guidance:** Invest in at least one scarf you like that accessorizes with your dressier clothes. As much as you love your baseball cap, it might not pair as well with your cocktail party attire.

> ⋛ **Guidance:** Steer clear of silk scarves simply because they tend to slide right off a shaved head. I bought long cotton scarves that were warmer and easier to tie into interesting knots.

Wigs

Wigs are controversial. Some people just totally hate them or are freaked out by them. Others *love them* for the change in "look" they can bring.

⋟ **Guidance:** Purchase at least one high-quality wig that you can wear to important events if it feels like a hat or scarf would be too informal or too obviously CANCER related. Insurance will often cover part or all of the cost of the wig. If your policy won't, there are places like the American Cancer Society that will supply wigs to cancer patients who have financial need.

I did not wear my wig that often (maybe ten times over my six-month BALD period?) but when I needed it, I had it. For me, the wig was indispensable when I was going out and needed to be super dressed up (no baseball cap accessorizing). The wig came in handy when I would go to a performance like a ballet or symphony or out to a fancy meal. I found that folks simply glanced at my hair/wig and moved on, rather than focusing on why I was wearing a headscarf.

⋟ **Guidance:** Invest in one of each option (one hat, one scarf, one wig) and see what works for you. It is, and will be, personal. The key is to do whatever you can to make yourself feel as beautiful as you can during this time.

Other hair loss: eyebrows, eyelashes, and "the unmentionables"

Eyebrows and eyelashes

If you lose your head hair, you're probably going to lose your eyebrows and eyelashes. Initially it is super weird because suddenly you're getting stuff (like lotion and dust) in your eyes that doesn't normally get in because you have eyelashes to keep it out.

> **Guidance:** Go to Sephora or the MAC counter or just about any make up counter at a department store, and ask the person working there to teach you how to draw on eyebrows. Armed with a brown eyebrow pencil and a small mirror, I started drawing my eyebrows on daily. I even had one person say to me "Well, at least you haven't lost your eyebrows!"

> **Guidance:** If/when you want to start encouraging your eyebrows and eyelashes to grow back in, you can invest in an eyelash growth serum like RevitaLash® or WooLash® or any of the other growth serums out there. They work.

"The unmentionables"

Yes, you lose hair over your entire body. Some people pay good money to get a "Brazilian" wax to remove their pubic hairs. You get it for free with your chemotherapy. And yes, it does feel different; in some cases, maybe it might even enhance your experience. I mean, there's got to be SOME upside with this whole cancer thing, right?

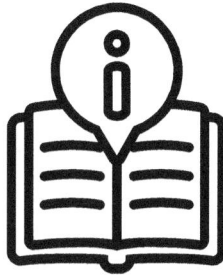

Chapter 12

Living with Cancer

The Cancer Companion

"The difference between you and me is that we both know we're going to die. But you actually believe it." My friend Bonnie said this to me when I was first diagnosed. She was right.

Most of us, prior to a major health revelation, believe we are invincible. Sickness and death are subjects to be considered in the future, and likely (if we're being honest with ourselves), experienced by *other* people. Not us.

In many ways, I have thought of that moment when I heard "You have cancer" as a demarcation line in my life. Now I see life as the *time before my diagnosis* and the *time after my diagnosis*.

If you are newly diagnosed, it is probably hard to imagine a time when you won't be completely stressed out by the fact that you have cancer. But if you make it through your treatments (and let's just both agree that you will), you will return to your life. And you will be changed.

As both Susan Sontag and Suleika Jaouad have written so beautifully, there are two kingdoms where we live. The kingdom of the well and the kingdom of the sick. When you live in the kingdom of the well, you cannot imagine what it is like to live in the kingdom of the sick. And once you are in the kingdom of the sick, you cannot imagine how you will ever get back to the kingdom of the well.

But I am hopeful that you will. And I am hopeful that you will learn to live peacefully with your life now that cancer has entered your kingdom. Your cancer diagnosis will earn you the right to annual/bi-annual scans and tests, and the hope each time to hear the magical words, "We see no evidence of disease."

It is hard living with the knowledge that you have (or had) cancer. It can haunt you if you let it. I don't have an easy answer for you here, but I will share with you how I try to think about it.

When I was first diagnosed and worked up the courage to send out a message to all of those I loved, I wrote this answer to the question everyone was asking us:

How you can help us

We need your unconditional love and constant prayers to whatever higher power you believe in. We need you to listen and to discuss this most scary topic with us, but also to talk with us about subjects *not* related to cancer. We're exhausted from the "all-cancer-all-the-time" channel we've been tuned into. We understand we're going to be living with cancer for the rest of our lives together, but we'd like to focus on the LIVING part of that statement, not the CANCER part of that statement.

Whatever comes, I hope that you can focus on the living part of your life.

I know it is controversial to say – but my year of cancer wasn't all bad.

Yes, I get that since my outcome was good (I lived), perhaps it colors my evaluation of the year. I am sure it does. But I think it is also because good stuff did happen that year that impacts the way I live now. Here are some of the big things I changed as I stepped into living my life, post-cancer:

I chose my life over my work

The work I did was central to my identity for decades. I loved what I did and I think I was good at it. And it is not that the work I do is no longer important to me—it is. It is simply a lower priority when compared to the people in my life. And it was for that reason that after my leave of absence to write a book, I made the extremely difficult decision to leave eBay. At its essence, eBay's mission is to enable economic opportunity for all. That mission is/was good and true and worth working for during the fourteen years I spent at eBay. I believed that mission to the core of my being.

And my God I felt I owed so much to the good people of eBay for their AMAZING support of me during my year of cancer! But after Geoff and I moved to Marin County, my commute became two hours each way on a good day. It was simply too much time out of my day and too far from the people I loved most...so I quit. I chose my life over my work. In the work/life balance conundrum, I continue to clearly and intentionally choose my life.

I committed to saying what is in my heart

For most of my life, I have been described as "outspoken." I have said what is on my mind. What I haven't always done is said what is in my heart. This sometimes takes a tremendous amount of courage depending on what it is I have needed to say and to whom. But I now reason that if my time is short, I want to ensure I am not leaving things unsaid. This means I say aloud when my feelings are hurt, even if it is embarrassing to admit it. This means I challenge people I love dearly when I believe their actions are in conflict with their integrity. This means I have told people I work with (people I work with!) that I love them. It is a more vulnerable way to live but whew – I have found it is a truer way to live.

I decided to stop worrying about time

I am a total fangirl of Lin-Manuel Miranda. I have lost count of the number of times Geoff and I have watched Hamilton (and Encanto, for that matter). Any article that mentions Lin is immediately click-bait for me. He recently shared on Twitter that he was asked, "Why is there always a ticking clock in your shows?" to which he replied, "Because there is always a ticking clock!" Boy did that resonate with me. I lived most of my life with the sound of a distant ticking in my head – aware and haunted by the watches I wore (and collected) to keep on schedule. At the beginning of my year of cancer treatments, I took my watch off. At first it was because I worried I would leave it in the imaging room at Stanford. Better to keep it at home and safe. After a while, I noticed that without a watch I spent less time checking the time. My day became less driven by what time it was. I still had doctors' appointments to get to, but there was less time-related stress in my life. And I liked it. I now live my life without my watch. I figure if my time is short, I shouldn't spend it counting the minutes to my next appointment or deadline; I should spend my life leaning into the adventure of it.

I decided to have a baby

My husband Geoff and I had been pursuing fertility treatments when I was first diagnosed with salivary gland cancer. When I was diagnosed with my second cancer, breast cancer, we were told by my breast oncologist that the hormonal therapy I would be on for the next ten years would disqualify me from being able to carry a baby. It was really hard news to hear but perhaps the trade-off we would need to accept in order to keep my cancers at bay.

Two years after I finished cancer treatments, I had a check-up with my breast oncologist. The two-year checkup is a big deal/milestone with breast cancer. Getting to your two-, five-, and ten-year anniversaries post-breast cancer are big reasons to celebrate. At the end of this appointment, as we were all smiling and celebrating this first milestone, I shared with the doctor that Geoff and I were contemplating hiring a surrogate to help us have a baby.

The Cancer Companion

My breast oncologist congratulated me on this big decision and said "You know, there was recently a study conducted in Europe. They studied a group of Belgian and German women who had had breast cancer and were on Tamoxifen. These women individually took themselves off their Tamoxifen (against doctor's orders), got pregnant, had babies, and then went back on their hormonal therapy. And here's the thing – they didn't have higher incidences of cancer recurrence."

"Wait. What are you saying?" I asked.

"If you want to carry a baby...I'm pretty confident you can. We would monitor you throughout the pregnancy of course, but given the low level of aggression of your cancer, I think you could try."

It took some convincing for Geoff to agree to me going off my hormonal therapy for the year+ it would take to get pregnant, be pregnant, and breast feed, but he did. He said he wanted a guarantee that neither cancer would come back while I wasn't taking my hormonal therapy. I reminded him that we never had that guarantee. That for the rest of our lives, we would need to learn to live with the knowledge that either cancer could come back at any time.

But I argued that if my time was short, I wanted to live as intensely and fully as I could. I wanted the experience of being pregnant, of delivering a baby, and of nurturing an infant. In many ways it was a very selfish decision because it centered on the experiences I wished to have. I believed the physical and emotional transformation I would undergo in becoming a mother was something I did not want to miss.

Unquestionably, my cancer experience informed my new perspective on life – but having a child changed that life. Cancer and a child both taught me to be present for the here and now; don't wish days or weeks away because you are going through a tough time or you are anticipating an exciting event coming up. Be present. Live through it. Experience the challenging and the exciting, the bad and the good. Because there will be a whole lot of good – especially if you look for it.

The Cancer Companion

I am hopeful that you are able to learn to live with your cancer, that you are able to breathe through all of this. It is hard. It really is. I wish I could give you something to say or do that will magically eliminate the physical, mental, and emotional pain you may be feeling now and in the future. I have shared with you my guidance based upon my experience and I am so hopeful this has been helpful to you on your journey. And, as new age-y as it might seem, I do wish to send you the loving-kindness mantra that helped me calm down and focus during my treatments as you go through yours.

May you be happy,

May you be healthy,

May you be at peace.

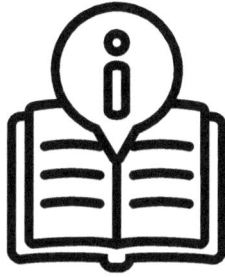

Appendix

Recommended Cancer Resources

American Cancer Society: (cancer.org)

This site has a tremendous amount of information about cancer, as well as services for cancer patients (like free rides to appointments, housing during treatment and a 1-800 phone line for questions). It is my go-to resource.

American Society of Clinical Oncology: (asco.org)

This is a patient information website developed to be the "voice of the world's cancer physicians." Everything is explained in super easy terms. They cover symptoms, treatment options, statistics, clinical trials. As the site says "Well-informed patients are their own best advocates and invaluable partners for physicians."

Cancer and Careers: (cancerandcareers.org)

This is a tremendous organization that helps cancer patients think about how to manage their cancer treatments with their work.

It has super helpful resources such as webinars/booklets/lists of organizations who provide support for those undergoing cancer treatment.

Cancer Prevention and Treatment Fund: (stopcancerfund.org)

This site is related to the National Center for Health Research. It has really interesting articles on cancer and treatments.

National Cancer Institute: (cancer.gov)

This is the federal government's primary cancer research organization. It is part of the National Institute of Health (NIH). Their site has a ton of information about cancer and its treatment.

National Comprehensive Cancer Network Guidelines for Patients: (nccn.org)

Site where you can look up clinical trials. This is a membership site but they have a patient section that is free.

Answering "How can I help?"

> Drive with me to appointments
> Take notes during my appointments
> Deliver food to me (especially ice cream)
> Drop off/pick up my kids from school
> Take my kids for a sleepover
> Walk my dog
> Mow my lawn/weed my garden
> Clean my house/send a cleaning service in
> Do my laundry/send the laundry out to a service
> Take me out to a meal/museum/movie/sports event/shopping
> Get me a gift certificate for a massage or spa
> Send me flowers
> Send me books/magazines/music/movies (especially if they are funny)
> Create a "chemo care package" for me complete with warm socks, a hat, trashy magazines (*People*, not porn), adult coloring books; whatever would be distracting for a couple of hours while

I sit in the infusion center.

⋛ Take a walk with me and discuss cancer

⋛ Take a walk with me and DON'T discuss cancer

⋛ Sit with me/hold my hand/hug me

Thank yous

Writing a book is a whole lot like sausage-making. It is oftentimes not pretty and unfortunately, if you want the book to be the best it can be – you need to have other (more objective) people read it and give their honest opinions. I got super lucky that the following people were willing to read my many shitty-first-drafts and tell me how I could make it better. Thank you to Jessie Becker, Rebecca Bloom, August Graves, Sarah Hoyt, John Lake, Sally Madsen, Deanna McDonald, Kenny Pate, and Nancy Svendsen. This was always the book I wanted to write and you brought tremendous insight and love to these pages and their guidance. Thank you.

I have found that until you have a deadline – you will always prioritize everything else above your goal. Thank you so much to Maria Olson of the American Cancer Society for your encouragement and for giving me that deadline. I am, in fact, so grateful to your entire team (especially Daniel Widner, Julia Gray, Cory Goodale, Rosa Navas, Staci Calvert, and Blythe Mooney). Thank you for including me on your extended team.

The Cancer Companion

A HUGE THANK YOU to Nanette Levin, my amazing editor. I am so appreciative of your dedication to making my work more crisp, more helpful, and more funny.

And finally, thank you to Geoff and to Rory. You are both ALWAYS my first priorities though recently you have had to endure me frantically typing on my computer even when I should be swimming in the resort pool with you. Don't worry. It's finished now and I am grabbing my sunscreen and towel. Meet you there.

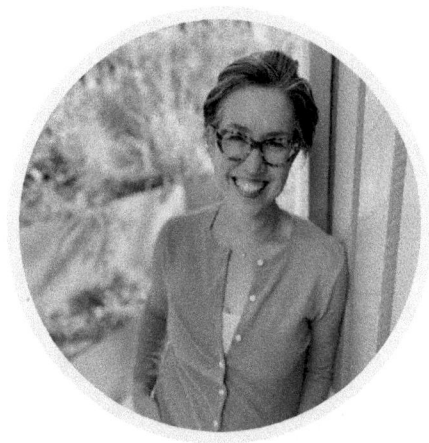

About The Author

Photo credit: Patti Lorin

Sarah E. McDonald lives in Mill Valley with her husband, Geoff, and daughter, Rory. Sarah has spent the majority of her 30-year career in the technology industry, 14 years of which were at eBay, where she was working when she was diagnosed with cancer. She now splits her time as an executive coach, workshop facilitator, keynote speaker, hopeful author, and fierce advocate for those undergoing cancer treatment. She raises money for rare cancer research through Memorial Sloan Kettering's Cycle for Survival and is a speaker and volunteer for the American Cancer Society.

Sarah received her MBA from Cornell University and her BA from Occidental College. Beyond cancer, Sarah is interested in all things people-related – especially when paired with food, wine, the outdoors, and/or music. Her first book, *The Cancer Channel: One year, Two cancers, Three miracles*, is a memoir focused on her experience being diagnosed with and treated for two cancers. *The Cancer Companion: A guide to getting your head and heart around your diagnosis and treatment* is her second book and is meant as a guidebook to those newly diagnosed with cancer.

Find out more about Sarah at **sarahemcdonald.com.**